STUDY GUIDE FOR NURSING PHARMACOLOGY

NORMA L. PINNELL, MSN, RN

College of Nursing
Southern Illinois University at Edwardsville
Edwardsville, Illinois

College of Nursing
Deaconess Health System
St. Louis, Missouri

MYRNA BRENNER WACKER, MS, RNC

College of Nursing
Southern Illinois University at Edwardsville
Edwardsville, Illinois

W.B. SAUNDERS COMPANY
A Division of Harcourt Brace & Company
Philadelphia London Toronto Montreal Sydney Tokyo

D1313684

W. B. Saunders Company
A Division of Harcourt Brace & Company
The Curtis Center
Independence Square West
Philadelphia, PA 19106-3399

Study Guide for Nursing Pharmacology

ISBN 0-7216-6783-X

Printed in the United States of America

Last digit is the print number: 9   8   7   6   5   4   3   2   1

Contributors

Lasca Beck, MS, RN
Nursing Liaison, Arizona State University West; Faculty Associate, Arizona State University, Tempe, Arizona

Elizabeth Ann Coleman, PhD, RNP
Associate Professor, College of Nursing, and Program Leader, Women's Oncology, Arkansas Cancer Research Center, University of Arkansas for Medical Sciences, Little Rock, Arkansas

Susan Grinslade, MSN, RN
Associate Professor, Jewish Hospital College of Nursing and Allied Health, St. Louis, Missouri

Gail Estock Haller, MS, RN
Assistant Professor, Division of Nursing, McKendree College, Lebanon, Illinois

Donna Henry, MSN, RN
Instructor of Nursing, Illinois Eastern Community Colleges, Olney, Illinois

Pamela E. Hugie, MSN, RN
Assistant Professor, Weber State University, Ogden, Utah

Kathy M. Ketchum, MS, RN
Doctoral Student and Research Assistant, St. Louis University, St. Louis, Missouri

Joan M. Kulpa, EdD, MSN, RN
Associate Professor, Nursing, Bradley University, Peoria, Illinois

Sandra Lindquist, MEd, MSN, RN
Associate Professor, Barnes College of Nursing, University of Missouri-St. Louis, St. Louis, Missouri

Jean Nelson, MEd, MSN, RN
Clinical Assistant Professor, Barnes College of Nursing, University of Missouri-St. Louis, St. Louis, Missouri

Marguerite Newton, PhD, RN
Assistant Professor, Southern Illinois University at Edwardsville, School of Nursing, Edwardsville, Illinois

Janet D. Pierce, DSN, RN, CCRN
Assistant Professor, University of Kansas School of Nursing, Kansas City, Kansas

Julia Ann Raithel, MSN, RN
Assistant Professor, Deaconess College of Nursing, St. Louis, Missouri

Robyn Rice, MS, RN
Associate Clinical Professor, Barnes College of Nursing, University of Missouri-St. Louis; Medical-Surgical Clinical Nurse Specialist, Family Services and Visiting Nurse Association, Alton, Illinois

Linda Ruholl, MS, RNC
Nursing Instructor and Pharmacology Instructor, Lake Land College, Mattoon, Illinois

Terry L. Seaton, PharmD, BCPS
Assistant Professor, St. Louis College of Pharmacy; Clinical Pharmacist, Department of Family Medicine, St. John's Mercy Medical Center, St. Louis, Missouri

Martha A. Spies, MSN, RN
Assistant Professor, Deaconess College of Nursing, St. Louis, Missouri

Janet L. Melnik Stewart, MNEd, RN
Nursing Instructor, The Western Pennsylvania Hospital School of Nursing, Pittsburgh, Pennsylvania

Carol M. Viamontes, MSN, RN
Clinical Nurse Specialist, Maternal-fetal Medicine, St. Mary's Health Center, St. Louis, Missouri

Joan Domigan Wentz, MSN, RN
Assistant Professor, Jewish Hospital College of Nursing and Allied Health, St. Louis, Missouri

Sharee A. Wiggins, MSN, RN, CRNI
Clinical Assistant Professor, Critical Care, University of Kansas School of Nursing, Kansas City, Kansas

Linda Nattkemper York, MSN, RN
Instructor, Barnes College of Nursing, University of Missouri-St. Louis, and Consultant, Independence Center, St. Louis, Missouri

INTRODUCTION FOR STUDENTS

Pharmacology may be a difficult topic for some students. The suggestions listed below are designed to make study of this topic easier.

1. Always complete the required readings before coming to class. Focus on content that describes either the drug category or classification and the prototype drug.

2. As you read, look up the definition of terms. This increases your comprehension of medical terminology and makes future study in all courses much easier.

3. Since abbreviations are used in tables to describe therapeutic dosages and schedules, make certain that you have a list of common abbreviations with your pharmacology notes.

4. Taking notes in class is easier when you are familiar with the drugs, terms, and diseases being discussed. You are able to listen to what is being **said** by the instructor instead of simply writing down words.

5. After class, review your notes and the reading material on the topics presented in class. At this time you can add important information from the book to your lecture notes if necessary.

6. After reviewing your notes and reading material, note any concepts or content that remains unclear. Clarify this material with your instructor.

7. Complete activities in the study guide that are appropriate for material being studied. Use these exercises to test your knowledge of the information and further identify areas that are unclear. A variety of different activities are offered for each chapter. Select those that are the most helpful to you.

TABLE OF CONTENTS

UNIT I   ORIENTATION TO PHARMACOLOGY

1. Introduction to Pharmacology 1
2. Legal Foundations of Pharmacologic Practice 4

UNIT II   GENERAL PRINCIPLES OF PHARMACOLOGY

3. Pharmaceutic Phase 7
4. Pharmacokinetic Phase 11
5. Pharmacodynamic Phase 15
6. Individual Variation in Drug Response 18
7. Drug Interactions 22

UNIT III   DRUG THERAPY AND THE NURSE

8. Drug Therapy and the Nursing Process 25

UNIT IV   THE INDIVIDUAL AND DRUG THERAPY

9. Cultural Influence on Drug Therapy 29
10. Psychosocial Factors Affecting Drug Therapy 32
11. Self-treatment 35
12. Substance Abuse and Addiction 38
13. Drug Therapy in Childbearing and Breastfeeding Clients 43
14. Drug Therapy in the Neonate and Pediatric Client 47
15. Drug Therapy in the Elderly Client 50
16. Nurse's Role in Drug Therapy in the Home 54

UNIT V   DRUGS AFFECTING THE CENTRAL NERVOUS SYSTEM

17. Overview of the Central Nervous System 57
18. Sedatives, Hypnotics, and Anxiolytics 61
19. Opioid and Nonopioid Analgesics 65
20. Psychotherapeutic Drugs 69
21. Antiepileptic Drugs 74
22. Central Nervous System Stimulants 78
23. Drugs Used to Treat Parkinson's Disease 82
24. Anesthetic Agents 88

UNIT VI   DRUGS AFFECTING THE AUTONOMIC NERVOUS SYSTEM

25. Overview of the Autonomic Nervous System 91
26. Drugs Affecting the Parasympathetic Nervous System 94
27. Drugs Affecting the Sympathetic Nervous System 99
28. Skeletal Muscle Relaxants 103

UNIT VII   DRUGS AFFECTING THE CARDIOVASCULAR SYSTEM

29. Overview of the Cardiovascular System 106
30. Drugs that Affect Vascular Tone 110
31. Cardiac Glycosides 113
32. Antiarrhythmic Drugs 117
33. Antihypertensive Drugs 120
34. Drugs Affecting Plasma Lipids and Coagulation Factors 125

UNIT VIII   DRUGS AFFECTING THE RENAL SYSTEM

35. Overview of the Renal System 129
36. Diuretics 131
37. Hyperuricemic Drugs 135

UNIT IX   DRUGS AFFECTING THE ENDOCRINE SYSTEM

38. Overview of Endocrine System 138
39. Drugs Used to Regulate Blood Glucose Levels 142
40. Drugs Affecting Hypothalamic and Pituitary Functions 147
41. Drugs Affecting Thyroid and Parathyroid Functions 151
42. Adrenal Corticoids 155

UNIT X   DRUGS AFFECTING THE RESPIRATORY SYSTEM

43. Overview of the Respiratory System 161
44. Nasal Decongestants, Antitussives, and Mucolytics 164
45. Bronchodilating Drugs and Related Agents 168

UNIT XI   DRUGS AFFECTING THE GASTROINTESTINAL SYSTEM

46. Overview of the Digestive System 172
47. Drugs Affecting the Upper Gastrointestinal Tract 177
48. Drugs Affecting the Lower Gastrointestinal Tract 182

UNIT XII   DRUGS AFFECTING THE BODY'S DEFENSE SYSTEM

49. Overview of Biologic Defense Mechanisms 187
50. Histamine-Receptor Agonists and Antagonists 191
51. Nonsteroidal, Anti-inflammatory Drugs 194
52. Immunosuppressant and immunostimulant Drugs 199
53. HIV Therapy 206

UNIT XIII   ANTIMICROBIAL DRUGS

54. Principles of Antimicrobial Therapy 209
55. Antibiotics 213
56. Urinary Tract Antiseptics 218
57. Antimycobacterial Drugs 222

58. Antifungal Drugs 225
59. Antiviral Drugs 228
60. Antiparasitic Drugs 231

UNIT XIV DRUGS AFFECTING THE REPRODUCTIVE SYSTEM

61. Overview of Female and Male Reproductive Systems 235
62. Drugs Affecting the Female Reproductive System 237
63. Drugs Affecting the Male Reproductive System 240

UNIT XV DRUGS AFFECTING THE SENSORY SYSTEM

64. Drugs Used in Ocular Disorders 243
65. Ear Preparations 246
66. Local Anesthesia 249

UNIT XVI DRUGS AFFECTING THE INTEGUMENTARY SYSTEM

67. Drugs Used to Treat Dermatologic Conditions 252

UNIT XVII DRUGS USED TO TREAT NEOPLASTIC DISEASES

68. Overview of Normal and Neoplastic Cell Growth 256
69. Antineoplastic Drugs 259

UNIT XVIII DRUGS FOR FLUID, ELECTROLYTE, AND NUTRITIONAL BALANCE

70. Fluid, Electrolyte, and Nutritional Balance 262
71. Fat-Soluble Vitamins 264
72. Water-Soluble Vitamins 268
73. Minerals 272
74. Agents Affecting the Volume and Ion Content of Body Fluids 275
75. Enteral and Parenteral Nutritional Therapy 279

UNIT XIX MISCELLANEOUS DRUG CATEGORIES

76. Antiseptics, Disinfectants, and Sterilants 282
77. Drugs Used to Manage Poisoning 284
78. Drugs Used for Diagnostic Procedures 286

ANSWER KEYS 289

CHAPTER 1
INTRODUCTION TO PHARMACOLOGY

DEFINITION OF TERMS

Define the following:

1. chemical name

2. drug

3. generic name

4. nonproprietary name

5. official name

6. pharmacognosy

7. pharmacopeia

8. pharmacy

9. proprietary name

10. prototype

HISTORIC PERSPECTIVE

Fill in the blanks on the following time line.

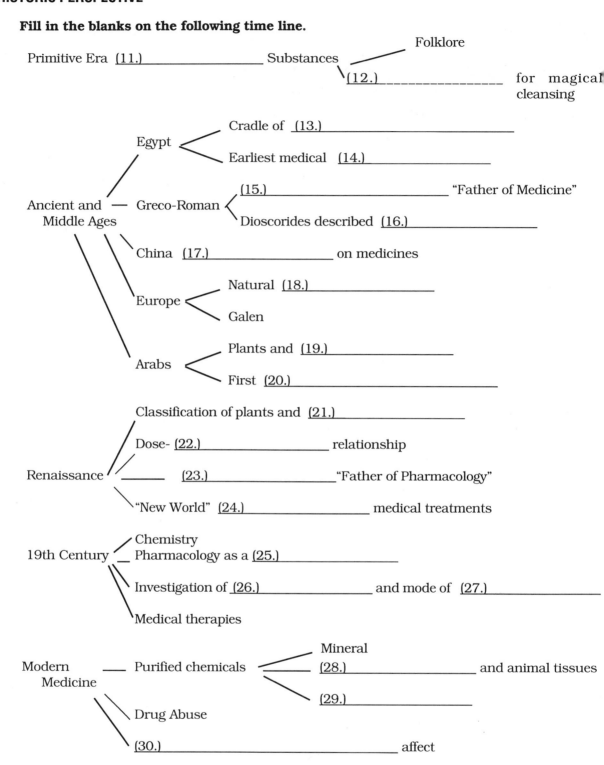

Primitive Era (11.)_____ Substances

Folklore

(12.)_____ for magical cleansing

Ancient and Middle Ages — Egypt

Cradle of (13.)_____

Earliest medical (14.)_____

Greco-Roman

(15.)_____ "Father of Medicine"

Dioscorides described (16.)_____

China (17.)_____ on medicines

Europe

Natural (18.)_____

Galen

Arabs

Plants and (19.)_____

First (20.)_____

Renaissance

Classification of plants and (21.)_____

Dose- (22.)_____ relationship

_____ (23.)_____ "Father of Pharmacology"

"New World" (24.)_____ medical treatments

19th Century

Chemistry

Pharmacology as a (25.)_____

Investigation of (26.)_____ and mode of (27.)_____

Medical therapies

Modern Medicine — Purified chemicals

Mineral

(28.)_____ and animal tissues

(29.)_____

Drug Abuse

(30.)_____ affect

MULTIPLE CHOICE

Select the best answer.

31. Which statement is most accurate about the chemical name of a drug?
    A. The letters USP are placed after the drug's name.
    B. It is the same as the generic name.
    C. It is a capitalized name that is owned by the drug manufacturer.
    D. It is a complex name that identifies the chemical structure of the drug.

32. Which statement regarding generic drugs is correct? Generic drugs

    A. cannot be patented with the U.S.
    B. must have the same dosage and route of administration as the approved drug product.
    C. must be proven to be clinically equivalent to the approved drug product.
    D. must have the same active ingredients, fillers, and additives as the approved drug product.

CRITICAL THINKING ACTIVITY

The home health nurse is assessing a new client who frequently changes physicians. The client has a bottle of unlabeled tablets that she has been taking. She states that the tablets were prescribed by a physician that no longer treats her. She does not know the name of the drug nor why the drug was prescribed. What steps would the nurse take in determining the drug's name, action, and therapeutic purpose?

CHAPTER 2
LEGAL FOUNDATIONS OF PHARMACOLOGIC PRACTICE

DEFINITION OF TERMS

Define the following:

1. investigational drug

2. legend

3. nonprescription

4. orphan drug

5. prescription

Match the law/act in Column A with the appropriate definition in Column B.

| Column A | Column B |

6. _____   Federal Pure Food and Drug Act (1906)

7. _____   Harrison Narcotic Act (1914)

8. _____   Federal Food, Drug, and Cosmetic Act (1938)

9. _____   Durham-Humphrey Amendment (1952)

10. _____   Kefauver-Harris Amendment (1962)

A.   required proof of efficacy and safety before marketing

B.   established labeling requirements and required drug toxicity studies

C.   established 2 categories of drugs

D.   restricted sale and manufacture of drugs

E.   attempted to regulate importation and marketing of narcotic drugs

F.   regulated labeling

Using the Controlled Drug Schedule identify the drug schedule for the following:

| Drug | Schedule |

11   terpin hydrate with codeine   _____

12.   paregoric   _____

13.   anabolic steroids   _____

14.   heroin   _____

15.   morphine   _____

16.   diazepam   _____

17.   mescaline   _____

18.   opium   _____

Match the Drug Developmental Phase in Column A with the appropriate description in Column B.

| Column A | Column B |

19. _____   Phase I

20. _____   Phase II

21. _____   Phase III

22. _____   Phase IV

A.   drug released for marketing

B.   double-blind, controlled studies are conducted

C.   testing involves 75 to 150 human volunteers; results in baseline data

D.   research done on drug's therapeutic effectiveness for a particular disease

MULTIPLE CHOICE

Select the best answer.

23. The legislation that resulted in standards for drug safety and efficacy was

   A.   Controlled Substance Act of 1970.
   B.   Durham-Humphrey Amendment of 1952.
   C.   Kefauver-Harris Act of 1962.
   D.   Drug Regulation and Reform Act of 1978.

24. Which of the following statements by a client involved in a drug research study would indicate lack of informed consent?

   A.   "I was so sleepy when the doctor explained this drug to me. What do you call it?"
   B.   "I am to keep a log of how I feel after I take this drug."
   C.   "This drug makes my mouth dry. The doctor said it would."
   D.   "I haven't has any leg cramps so far. The doctor told me to watch for them."

25. Phase I studies are conducted for:

   A.   toxicity evaluation in animals.
   B.   initial pharmacologic evaluation.
   C.   limited controlled evaluation.
   D.   extended clinical evaluation.

CRITICAL THINKING ACTIVITY

Discuss the FDA drug testing requirements in light of the concerns over the HIV epidemic. What are the ethical considerations involved in speeding up drug approval for treatment of this disease?

CHAPTER 3

PHARMACEUTIC PHASE

DEFINITION OF TERMS

Complete the sentences, choosing the correct term for each defintion.

alkaloids, glycosides, gums, oils, pharmaceutic phase, resins, disintegration, dissolution, active ingredient, excipient

Complex semisolid or solid substances of plant origin that are insoluble in water are

1. _____.

Inert substances that form the bases of drugs are

2. _____.

Compounds that are composed of sugar units, usually glucose, and nonsugar components are

3. _____.

The actual breakdown of a dosage form in the aqueous contents of the digestive tract is

4. _____.

Plant exudates that are polysaccharides are

5. _____.

Highly viscous volatile or fixed liquids that are the liquid form of lipids are

6. _____.

Entering a solution as solute particles is

7. _____.

Organic chemical compounds composed of carbon, hydrogen, nitrogen, and oxygen that are usually specific to a given plant species are

8. _____.

The components of drugs responsible for producing their actions are

9. _____.

Information on sources of drugs, constituents of drug products, formulation of drugs, routes of administration, drug stability, and drug storage are included in the

10. _____.

SOURCES OF DRUGS

Match the drug source in Column A with the appropriate description in Column B

Column A	Column B

Column A

11. ____   Alkaloid

12. ____   Glycosides

13. ____   Gums

14. ____   Resins

15. ____   Fixed oils

16. ____   Volatile oils

Column B

A.   An exudate that swells when water is added.

B.   Substance that is greasy and does not evaporate easily.

C.   Form water-soluble salts when combined with acids.

D.   Substance with a pleasant odor and taste that evaporates easily.

E.   Substance with sugar that increases solubility, absorption, permeability, and distribution.

F.   Amorphous exudates that are insoluble in water.

Multiple Choice

DRUG ROUTES

Select the best answer.

17. Which statement is most accurate about drug routes?
    A.   Topically administered drugs produce only local effects.
    B.   The major systemic routes involve the lymphatic or vascular system.
    C.   The oral route is the best route to use for systemic drug delivery.
    D.   The major routes for systemic effect are oral and enteral.

18. Which answer is correct about parenteral drug routes?
    A.   Subcutaneous injection involves injection into or just under the skin layer.
    B.   Intrathecal drugs are administered directly into a joint.
    C.   Parenteral drug routes involve injection or infusion into any part of the body.
    D.   Intravenous drugs are infused directly into the vascular system.

19. Which sentence best describes parenteral drug routes?
    A.   The intravenous route provides the most rapid, predictable drug delivery.
    B.   The intraarterial route is frequently used to test for allergies.
    C.   The principle sites for intramuscular injection are the rectus and deltoid muscles.
    D.   The intraspinal route goes directly into the subarachnoid or subdural space.

20. Which choice is most appropriate about topical routes of drug administration?
    A.   Buccal administration involves holding drugs under the tongue while they dissolve.
    B.   Sublingual drugs are absorbed by blood vessels and circulated through the body.
    C.   Instillation involves administering drugs to diffuse through the skin.
    D.   Rectally instilled drugs absorb at the same rate and extent as oral drug, since both are absorbed into the gastrointestinal tract.

STUDY QUESTIONS

DRUG PREPARATION, STABILITY, AND STORAGE

21. Why is it important to keep solutions stored in containers with tight fitting caps?

22. What are two important details about preparing suspensions?

23. Why isn't crushing recommended for coated tablets or sustained release tablets?

24. Why shouldn't the nurse use any remaining medication after withdrawing the desired dose from an ampule?

25. What should the nurse add to a vial before withdrawing the medication?

26. What usually suggests deterioration in liquid dosage forms?

27. What usually suggests deterioration in solid dosage forms?

28. What are four important storage factors that can alter the effectiveness of drugs?

CRITICAL THINKING ACTIVITY

The home health nurse is working with an elderly female client on a fixed income. The client stores her medications on a shelf above the stove. When the nurse checks the medication, he finds that some of the tablets have disintegrated. The client says that she will just mix them in with juice because they are so expensive. She says she cannot afford to discard them and buy new ones. What should this nurse do?

CHAPTER 4
PHARMACOKINETIC PHASE

DEFINITION OF TERMS

Define the following:

1. affinity

2. bioavailability

3. blood-brain barrier

4. competitive binding

5. drug reservoirs

6. enterohepatic recycling

7. first-pass phenomenon

8. loading dose

9 maintenance dose

10. metabolites

11. nonspecific binding

12. pharmacokinetic

13. placental barrier

14. plasma half-life

15. plasma-protein binding

16. plateau principle

17. solubility

18. therapeutic index

19. Develop a drawing that depicts the four pharmacokinetic processes. Describe each process.

Match the terms in Column A with the appropriate definition in Column B.

Column A	Column B

20. ____	passive diffusion	A.	movement through membrane pores from area of highest to area of lowest concentration
21. ____	active transport		
22. ____	pinocytosis	B.	cell membrane surrounds and engulfs substance
23. ____	filtration	C.	movement of molecules across cell membrane against concentration gradient
		D.	random movement of drug molecules from place of highest drug concentration to place of lowest concentration

Indicate if the statement is true or false. Correct the false statements.

24. ____ A drug must be attached to a plasma protein in order to cross the cell membrane.

25. ____ Water soluble drugs cross the blood-brain barrier easily.

26. ____ Enzymes capable of biotransformation are found in all body tissues.

27. ____ Low serum concentrations of free-unbound drug accelerates absorption.

28. ____ Ionized drugs do not diffuse across lipid membranes easily.

29. ____ The microsomal enzyme system of the kidneys is responsible for metabolizing most drugs.

30. ____ Most drugs are excreted through the renal system.

STUDY QUESTIONS

31. Describe 5 factors that alter oral drug absorption.

32. Describe the impact of cardiac output on drug distribution.

33. Describe how ethnic differences alter biotransformation.

34. Chart a time-response curve for a drug using the following parameters: onset of action 30 minutes; time to peak effect 1.5 hours, an duration of action 4 hours.

MULTIPLE CHOICE

Select the best answer.

35. Which of the following best defines biotransformation?
    A.   differential distribution of a drug
    B.   binding of a drug to plasma protein
    C.   metabolic conversion of a foreign substance
    D.   therapeutic effect of a drug

36. A client has a drug serum level of 100 units/ml. The drug's half-life is 1 hour. If concentrations above 20 units/ml are toxic and no additional drug is administered, what is the minimum time that it will take for serum levels to reach the nontoxic range?
    A.   1 to 2 hours
    B.   2 to 3 hours
    C.   3 to 4 hours
    D.   4 to 5 hours

CRITICAL THINKING ACTIVITY

The nurse is administering an oral analgesic to a malnourished 69-year-old male. The client was admitted with pain in his left hip and chronic renal failure. Name four variables in the situation that may influence drug action. Briefly explain how each variable alters drug action.

CHAPTER 5
PHARMACODYNAMIC PHASE

DEFINITION OF TERMS

Define the following:

1. agonist

2. antagonist

3. antimetabolites

4. dose-response curve

5. drug-enzyme interaction

6. drug-receptor interaction

7. drug potency

8. efficacy

9. pharmacodynamics

10 structurally nonspecific

11. structurally specific

Indicate if the statement is true or false. Correct the false statements.

12. ____ Drugs that physically modify the cell's environment do not change specific cellular functions.

13. ____ Drugs that produce their effects by interacting with enzymes are considered structurally nonspecific drugs.

14. ____ Affinity describes the drug's propensity to be a given receptor site.

15. ____ An agonist is a drug that has the ability to initiate a desired therapeutic effect.

16. ____ Drug efficacy refers to the relative amount of a drug required to produce the desired response.

17. ____ The relationship between the drug dose administered and the response generated is the therapeutic index.

18. Diagram the interaction of a drug with a receptor site. Using the diagram explain the terms affinity, efficacy, agonist, and antagonist to a class mate.

STUDY QUESTIONS

19. Differentiate between competitive antagonists and non-competitive antagonists.

20. Distinguish between drug action and drug effects.

21. Describe how circadian rhythms affect the pharmacodynamic phase.

22. Determine the therapeutic index based on the following information: pain relief occurs at a dose of 10 mg and lethal dose is 250 mg.

Multiple Choice

Select the best answer.

23. A cardiac glycoside has been prescribed for the client. When explaining the action of the drug, the nurse is explaining what aspect of drug therapy?
A. pharmacotherapeutics
B. pharmacodynamics
C. pharmacokinetics
D. pharmacognostics

24. The lethal-dose 50% (LD50) of a drug informs the nurse about the average dose needed to :
A. produce desired therapeutic effects in 50 % of the individuals treated.
B. cause 50% of the known undesired clinical responses.
C. cause toxicity in 50% of the individuals treated.
D. produce minimum therapeutic effects.

CRITICAL THINKING ACTIVITY

Why is it accurate to state that pharmacologic antagonists don't cause effects but allow effects to occur?

CHAPTER 6
INDIVIDUAL VARIATION IN DRUG RESPONSE

DEFINITION OF TERMS

Match the term with the correct definition.

1. ____ Pharmacogenetics

2. ____ Adverse reactions

3. ____ Side effects

4. ____ Toxic effects

5. ____ Intolerance

6. ____ Drug allergy

7. ____ Idiosyncratic responses

8. ____ Tolerance

9. ____ Cumulative effects

10. ____ Dependence

11. ____ Summation

12. ____ Synergistic effect

13. ____ Potentiation

14. ____ Antagonistic effect

15. ____ Interaction

A. Unusual abnormal drug response caused by genetics

B. Physical or emotional craving for a drug.

C. Process of two or more entities acting on each other

D. The reaction of the body's immune system to the presence of a drug.

E. When administration of a second drug intensifies or prolongs the effect of the first drug.

F. The study of the genetic influences on responses to drugs.

G. Occurrence of side effects or adverse reactions to normal doses of a drug.

H. When the combined effect of two drugs is less than that of either one of the drugs alone.

I. Responses other that the expected clinical response that occur with normal drug doses.

J. Decreased response to a drug as a consequence of prior exposure.

K. Harmful effects from high doses or increased sensitivity to a drug.

L. Additive response when the combined effect of two drugs is equal to the sum of the effect of each drug administered alone.

M. The result of accumulation of a drug in the body.

N. Unwanted, undesired, and possible harmful side effects of drugs.

O. Occurs when the addition of a second drug results in a combined effect greater than the sum of the effects of each of the two drugs alone.

FACTORS AFFECTING INDIVIDUAL CLINICAL RESPONSES

List two examples of how response is altered for each factor affecting individual response to drugs:

16. Body size and weight
    Increased size=   Decreased size=

17. Gender
    Females=   Males=

18. Age
    Infants=   Elderly=

19. Genetics

20. Ethnicity

21. Pathophysiologic

22. Psychosocial

23. Nutritional

24. Environment

MULTIPLE CHOICE

UNDESIRED CLINICAL RESPONSE TO DRUG THERAPY

Select the best answer.

25. Which statement is most accurate about responses to drug therapy?
    A. Some drugs are prescribed for their beneficial side effects.
    B. A predictable adverse response is an anticipated effect of the drug.
    C. Drugs with narrow therapeutic indexes have a low potential for toxic effects.
    D. Undesired clinical responses are the result of careless testing and monitoring.

26. Which answer is correct about responses to single drug administration?
    A. Immediate hypersensitivity is sometimes called cell-mediated hypersensitivity.
    B. One example of delayed hypersensitivity is anaphylaxsis.
    C. Immediate hypersensitivity reactions are due to antibodies present from prior exposure.
    D. An example of immediate hypersensitivity is serum sickness.

27. Which sentence best describes other responses to single drug administration?
    A. Idiosyncratic responses usually involve altered drug metabolism.
    B. Metabolic tolerance is caused by a reduction in drug concentration at the receptor site, usually precipitated by increased biotransformation.
    C. Cellular tolerance causes the body to be unable to metabolize and excrete the drug, causing diminished effectiveness.
    D. Cross-tolerance is a desirable response because it means tolerance to one drug confers tolerance to another.

28. Which choice is most appropriate about response to combinations of drugs?
    A. The incidence of adverse reactions increases as the total number of prescribed drugs increases.
    B. Summative effects can only occur when drugs interact.
    C. Pharmacologic antagonism means the drug produces the pharmacologically opposite effect at the same sites.
    D. The antagonistic effect is always an adverse response to drugs.

29. Which statement is most accurate about iatrogenic responses?
    A. Iatrogenic responses are the result of drug-drug, drug-nutrient, and drug-environment interactions.
    B. The skin is the most commonly affected organ in the body.
    C. The kidneys are the first organs to receive the drug after it is absorbed by the intestine.
    D. The liver is at risk for damage from drugs because it has the highest blood supply and oxygen consumption in the body.

30. Which answer is correct about iatrogenic responses?
    A. Nephritis and nephropathy are toxic responses of the neurologic system to drugs.
    B. Teratogenesis describes toxic cardiac responses to drugs.
    C. Ocular toxicity and ototoxicity are usually mild iatrogenic responses.
    D. Blood dyscrasias are serious life threatening hematologic responses to drugs.

CLINICAL RESPONSE TO DRUG THERAPY

Fill in the blanks of the graphics. (check pages 47–50 in text book)

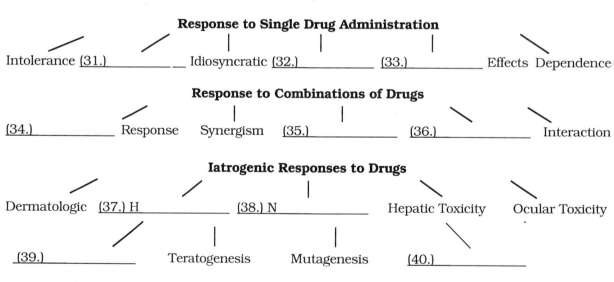

Response to Single Drug Administration

Intolerance (31.)_____ Idiosyncratic (32.)_____ (33.)_____ Effects   Dependence

Response to Combinations of Drugs

(34.)_____ Response   Synergism   (35.)_____ (36.)_____ Interaction

Iatrogenic Responses to Drugs

Dermatologic   (37.) H_____ (38.) N_____ Hepatic Toxicity   Ocular Toxicity

(39.)_____ Teratogenesis   Mutagenesis   (40.)_____

CRITICAL THINKING ACTIVITY

The nurse is assigned a client in the hospital that has just been prescribed to start anticoagulants and cardiac drugs. What are the primary responsibilities of the nurse in relation to client response to these drugs?

What are 5 steps the nurse should take if an undesirable reaction is assessed?

Chapter 7
DRUG INTERACTIONS

Definition of Terms

Define the following:

1. Drug-drug interaction

2. Drug-nutrient interaction

3. Drug-environment interaction

DRUG-DRUG INTERACTIONS

Fill in the blanks with the correct word or phrase.
Direct Physical or Chemical Interactions:

4. In a direct drug-drug interaction each drug is m_____.

5. Pharmacokinetic interactions alter the absorption, d_____ b_____, or excretion of drugs.

6. Usually a_____ drugs are excreted faster in a_____ urine.

7. Pharmacodynamic interactions result from the _____ _____

DRUG-NUTRIENT INTERACTIONS

Provide examples for each of the following.

8. Drugs that act as physical barrier to fat-soluble vitamins.

9.   Drugs that alter nutrient metabolism and utilization.

10.   Drugs that alter excretion of drugs.

11.   Drugs whose absorption rate is decreased by food.

12.   Food and drug combinations that are antagonistic.

13.   Drugs affected by the intake of alcohol.

14.   Drugs affected by the intake of tyramine.

Study Questions

15.   The nurse is administering oral pain medication to Mr. R., a malnourished 69 year old client with pain in his left hip and chronic renal failure. It is 6:00 P. M., and he just finished supper.

Identify four variables in the situation which may influence the drug action of the pain medication. Briefly explain why these variables will influence the drug action.

16.   Explain how antacids can decrease the effectiveness of certain drugs if administered concurrently with the drugs.

17.   Provide examples of two drugs that can alter the biotransformation of other drugs.

18. Describe the impact of the environment on drug therapy.

MULTIPLE CHOICE

CLINICAL IMPLICATIONS OF DRUG INTERACTIONS

Select the best answer.

19. Which sentence best describes pharmacokinetic interactions?
    A. Oral drugs most often interact to slow absorption of drugs in the stomach.
    B. The most common alteration in distribution has to do with ionization of drugs.
    C. Inhibiting biotransformation means inhibiting metabolism of drugs.
    D. Alterations in urinary pH usually increase the excretion of other drugs.

20. Which choice is most appropriate about clinical implications of drug interactions?
    A. Effective, safe use of drugs is the sole responsibility of the nurse.
    B. Interactions intensifying response increase the risk for adverse and toxic effects.
    C. Interactions usually intensify, rather than reducing the response.
    D. Multiple-drug therapy does not increase the risk of interaction.

CRITICAL THINKING ACTIVITY

The nurse is in a clinic setting where a diabetic client taking Orinase has received a new prescription for Edecrin, a diuretic. What steps should the nurse take to insure safe administration of the new drug?

Chapter 8
DRUG THERAPY AND THE NURSING PROCESS

Definition of Terms

Define the following:

1. Bolus

2. IV piggyback

3. IV push

4. Needle gauge

5. Needle length

Develop a drawing that depicts the nursing process. Describe each phase in the process.

Indicate if the statement is true or false. Correct the false statements.

6.   ____   Drugs are absorbed more rapidly intramuscularly than subcutaneously.

7.   ____   A 20 gauge needle is usually used for subcutaneous injections.

8.   ____   A vial usually contains only one dose of a drug.

9.   ____   When a drug is withdrawn from an ampule, an amount of air equal to the amount o
             solution to be withdrawn must be injected into the ampule.

10. ____   The use of oil as a vehicle for drugs markedly speeds up absorption of intramuscula
             injections

11. ____   Drugs in oily vehicles should not be administered intravenously.

Match the abbreviations in Column A with the correct answer in Column B.

Column A   **Column B**

12. ____   ac   A.   one half

13. ____   bid   B.   after meals

14. ____   PRN   C.   of each

15. ____   aa   D.   every day

16. ____   qd   E.   when required

17. ____   stat   F.   two times a day

18. ____   pc   G.   drop

19. ____   gtt   H.   right eye

20. ____   OD   I.   every hour

21. ____   qh   J.   before meals

22. ____   tid   K.   immediately

            L.   three times a day

STUDY QUESTIONS

23.   The type of needle selected for an intramuscular injection depends upon what factors?

24.   You encounter a new drug for which you have only the trade and generic names. How would you
      proceed to learn about the pharmacodynamic and pharmacokinetic properties of this drug?

25. A general guide to use in drug administration is the "five rights." Identify and describe each of the rights.

26. The primary care provider prescribes 750 mg PO of tetracycline. The drug is available in 250-mg capsules. How many capsules would you administer?

Multiple Choice

Select the best answer.

27. The physical assessment contains:
    A. subjective data.
    B. subjective and objective data.
    C. objective data.

28. The diagnosis, "High risk for injury related to diminished vision and fatigue associated with drug therapy" is written:
    A. incorrectly because both clauses say the same thing.
    B. correctly because the second clause explains the etiology of the diagnosis.
    C. incorrectly the identified response can not be altered.
    D. using legally inadvisable language.
    E. incorrectly because it contains a medical diagnosis.

29. Which of the following nursing diagnoses would be considered high priority based on Maslow's hierarchy?
    A. Altered body image related to ineffective coping with scar.
    B. Decreased activity tolerance related to cast on right leg.
    C. High risk for injury related to decreased vision.
    D. Impaired oxygenation related to increased respiratory secretions.

30. Which one of the following is an example of an expected outcome?
    A. Pulse 120, respirations 18, states she is ill.
    B. Client will increase his level of mobility.
    C. Susceptibility to injury.
    D. Client will eat 2000 calories a day by 10/12/96.

31. The amount of medication administered subcutaneously should not exceed:
    A. 0.5 ml.
    B. 1 ml.
    C. 2 ml.
    D. 5 ml.

32. When pouring liquid, the nurse should:
    A. hold the medicine glass at eye level while pouring.
    B. pour from the side of the bottle with the label.
    C. read the measurement at the highest point of the meniscus.
    D. place the medicine glass on the countertop while pouring.

CRITICAL THINKING ACTIVITY

You are collecting a drug history on a client who asks whether an equivalent generic drug would be an acceptable substitute for one of his prescribed drugs.

What immediate advice would you give this client?

What additional information might you need before advising the client further?

Chapter 9
CULTURAL INFLUENCE ON DRUG THERAPY

DEFINITION OF TERMS

Match the term with the correct definition.

1. _____ Acculturation

2. _____ Culture

3. _____ Culture shock

4. _____ Ethnicity

5. _____ Ethnocentrism

6. _____ Stereotyping

7. _____ Transcultural nursing

A. Feelings of bewilderment, confusion, and frustration when a person is confronted with an unfamiliar culture.

B. An area of study and practice focused on providing culturally appropriate nursing care.

C. The belief that one's own culture is superior to others.

D. Changing cultural practices to those of the dominant society.

E. Common biologic and/or physical characteristics of a group of people.

F. Common beliefs, customs, values, norms, behavioral patterns, and lifestyle practices of a group.

G. Viewing everyone of a certain culture as the same, without recognizing individual differences.

Fill in the blanks and list a cultural or ethnic example for each factor.

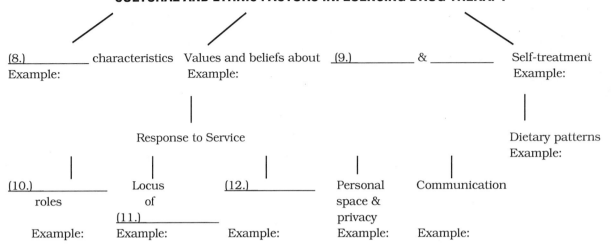

CULTURAL AND ETHNIC FACTORS INFLUENCING DRUG THERAPY

(8.)_____ characteristics   Values and beliefs about   (9.)_____ & _____   Self-treatment
Example: Example: Example:

Response to Service   Dietary patterns
                                                                                          Example:

(10.)_____   Locus   (12.)_____   Personal   Communication
   roles   of   space &
                  (11.)_____   privacy
   Example: Example: Example: Example: Example:

MULTIPLE CHOICE

Select the best answer.

13. Which statement is most accurate about transcultural nursing care?
    A. The purpose is to change client behavior.
    B. The purpose is to acculturate the client to the health care system.
    C. The purpose is to give more effective appropriate nursing care.
    D. The purpose is to find out more about different cultures.

14. Which answer is correct about how different cultures view each other?
    A. Culturally different people should adopt the practices of the dominant culture.
    B. Stereotyping is the disturbance people feel when exposed to unfamiliar cultures.
    C. Culture shock is the belief that your culture is superior.
    D. People can be unaware that they are ethnocentric.

15. Which sentence best describes cultural and ethnic differences?
    A. Cultures who have an internal locus of control will be more likely to engage in self-care practices.
    B. In some cultures, health care decisions may be made by someone besides the affected person.
    C. Touch and gestures are a universal language and can be used across cultures.
    D. Folk medicine is always harmful and should be discouraged.

16. Which choice is most appropriate about cultural assessment?
    A. Cultural sensitivity should begin with initial contact with client.
    B. The most important part of cultural assessment is following a recognized framework.
    C. Once you know the basic customs and practices of a culture, you can understand anyone from that culture.
    D. Clients from different cultural backgrounds usually describe the same symptoms for a particular health problem.

17. Which example best describes culturally appropriate nursing care?
    A. The nurse determines a client can understand English because they speak it.
    B. The nurse makes decisions about client care and then informs the client.
    C. The nurse incorporates all folk practices into the plan of care.
    D. The nurse has an understanding of his or her own cultural beliefs.

18. The purpose of learning about other cultural beliefs and practices is to:
    A. understand the practices of everyone from that cultural group.
    B. determine the beliefs that do not fit with scientific medicine.
    C. provide information on possible practices and beliefs to aid in assessment and appropriate care.
    D. learn how to treat people of that culture.

19. The nurse is demonstrating culturally appropriate care by:
    A. providing a translator of the same gender to discuss care.
    B. speaking loudly, slowly, and clearly to the client.
    C. explaining the reason why the hospital gown is open in the back.
    D. drawing a diagram of the times for medications to be taken.

20. Which statement is most accurate about cultural and ethnic variations?
    A. African-Americans usually lack a social support system.
    B. Timing of dosages after discharge may be a problem for Native Americans.
    C. Touch is usually important to Asian Americans.
    D. Most Hispanics value individualism.

21. The nurse is caring for a Hispanic client. What common cultural and ethnic variations should the nurse assess?
    A. A diet high in protein because it might affect drug response.
    B. Dislike of touch or close interpersonal distance.
    C. Belief in the Yin and Yang imbalance causing illness.
    D. Mistrust of culturally different health care providers.
    E. Direct.communication is preferred.

22. The nurse is caring for an Asian American client. What common cultural and ethnic variations should the nurse assess?
    A. Prayer is an important part of treatment.
    B. Eye contact is important.
    C. Lactose intolerance is often present.
    D. Self-expression of emotion is important.
    E. Individual decision making is valued.

CRITICAL THINKING ACTIVITY

You are a nurse on a busy hospital gynecology unit that has been assigned a client who is Hispanic. Other nurses inform you that the client is quite unreasonable and is driving everyone "crazy." The other nurses say that she nods in agreement to instructions for treatments, then doesn't follow them, that she will not discuss her gynecological problems with the doctors, that she becomes upset when the doctors want to examine her body, and that she always wants her family present, making the room crowded. What should your role be as a nurse in this case?

Chapter 10
PSYCHOSOCIAL FACTORS AFFECTING DRUG THERAPY

Definition of Terms

Fill in the blanks.

Behavior is an (1.)_____ response to environmental (2.)_____ and includes (3.)_____ reports about emotional state, (4.)_____, and thoughts.

Health behaviors are activities that influence health positively or (5.)_____that result from health (6.)_____.

Illness behavior is the (7.)_____of an individual to an (8.)_____.

Multiple Choice

Select the best answer.

9. What statement is most accurate about the Health Belief Model?
   A. It explains behaviors that enhance health, prevent illness or detect illness.
   B. It can be used to explain and predict health behaviors.
   C. It can be used to explain the client's health-wellness status.
   D. It can be used to assess the health and social resources available to a client.

10. According to the Health Belief Model, for a client to get a Td booster to prevent tetanus and diphtheria:
    A. He or she must know someone who has had either tetanus or diphtheria.
    B. There must be no barriers, such as finances, convenience, or pain to getting the immunization.
    C. He or she must have an internal locus of control for their health behavior.
    D. He or she must feel they are susceptible to becoming ill with either disease if they don't get the immunization.

11. Which answer is correct about understanding health behaviors?
    A. Patients who practice health-seeking behaviors usually are compliant with preventive treatments.
    B. Models of health behavior consider the medical model to examine the physiology of illness.
    C. The focus of the Human Ecologic Model is on environmental factors that influence health behaviors.
    D. The focus of the Resource Model of Preventive Behavior is on use of community health resources to prevent disease.

12. Which sentence best describes psychologic response to illness and drug therapy?
    A. The first stage of illness is assumption of the sick role.
    B. Clients usually respond in very similar ways to illness and drug therapy.
    C. Self-treatment usually occurs in the last two stages of illness.
    D. Denial of symptoms may cause delay in seeking care.

13. Which choice is most appropriate regarding psychological factors related to drug therapy?
    A. Placebos have been shown in studies to be ineffective to alleviate pain and sleeplessness.
    B. Past experience with drugs seldom influences current experiences.
    C. If a client does not expect positive responses from a drug, it is less likely to be effective.
    D. Physical symptoms do not usually occur from psychological responses to drugs.

14. Which type of behavior would indicate to a nurse that a client will probably be compliant with drug therapy?
    A. High self-esteem
    B. Internal locus of control
    C. Independence
    D. Dependence

15. Which answer is correct about psychosocial nursing considerations and the nursing process?
    A. The assessment should focus mostly on the physical response to drugs.
    B. Planning must be done solely by the nurse, since they have the expert knowledge.
    C. Interventions focus on involving the client in care and decision making.
    D. Evaluation should focus on expected physical outcomes from drug therapy.

STUDY QUESTIONS

16. List 3 fears related to drug therapy.

17. List 3 other feelings and their possible causes that clients and families may experience related to drug therapy.

18.   List 4 psychosocial factors to assess regarding client response to drug therapy.

19.   What would the nurse consider a negative response to drug therapy and compliance related to psychosocial factors?

CRITICAL THINKING ACTIVITY

You are a nurse in a home health agency. You are visiting a client after a week on a new drug. The client says he is experiencing all of the side effects you mentioned last week. You wonder if the client is suggestible and not really suffering from adverse effects of the drug. What should you do?

Chapter 11
SELF-TREATMENT

Definition of Terms

Complete the sentences, using the correct term for each definition.

Self-administration, self-medication, self-treatment, acupressure, acupuncture, herbalism, homeopathy.

1. _____ is the use of leaves, flowers, stems, or roots of plants to treat illness.

2. _____ is a noninvasive technique which applies pressure from the practitioner's fingers to acupuncture sites to cure or treat disease.

3. _____ is the act of properly and responsibly treating oneself with nonprescription drugs.

4. _____ is a system of therapeutics that treats disease with drugs capable of producing the same symptoms in healthy individuals as those of the ill person.

5. _____ is the use of prescribed drugs for other than prescribed purposes.

6. _____ is a technique that inserts needles into specific points in the body to relieve discomfort.

7. _____ is the practice of treating oneself with over-the-counter drugs.

Multiple Choice

Select the best answer.

8. Which statement is most accurate about self-care?
   A. It emphasizes that the individual is the object of health care.
   B. It emphasizes individuals taking responsibility for their own health.
   C. It emphasizes nontraditional medical practices.
   D. It emphasizes care of self during illness.

9. Which answer about self-treatment is correct?
   A. Self-medication is a part of self-treatment.
   B. Self-administration involves allowing clients to administer their own prescription drugs while hospitalized.
   C. Self-medication is never desirable.
   D. Self-care always involves self-medication.

10. Which sentence best describes use of OTC remedies?
    A. Their use is gradually decreasing with the increase of effective prescription drugs.
    B. These drugs are not as potent as prescription drugs.
    C. They are often used in the place of prescription drugs.
    D. Herbal remedies do not have any adverse effects with their use.

Below each factor briefly describe how it influences OTC drug use.

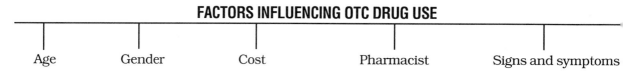

FACTORS INFLUENCING OTC DRUG USE

| Age | Gender | Cost | Pharmacist | Signs and symptoms |

STUDY QUESTIONS

11. List 3 reasons for the increase in self-care in the United States.

12. Discuss reasons why OTC drugs can be hazardous.

3.   Compile a list of OTC drugs that your family, including extended family take. Compare with one of your classmates lists.

4.   Make a list of all of the OTC drugs that you have taken in the last 5 years. Look these drugs up in a drug reference book and note side effects.

CRITICAL THINKING ACTIVITY

A client in the hospital with breast cancer discloses to you that she has been receiving acupuncture treatments which have helped her with the pain. What is your nursing responsibility?

CHAPTER 12
SUBSTANCE ABUSE AND ADDICTION

DEFINITION OF TERMS

Match the term with the correct definition.

1. _____ Circumstantial use
2. _____ Experimental phase
3. _____ Intensified use
4. _____ Social-recreational phase
5. _____ Substance abuse
6. _____ Addiction
7. _____ Compulsive phase
8. _____ Dependence
9. _____ Acetaldehyde
10. _____ Hash
11. _____ Hash oil
12. _____ Hallucinogens

A. When an individual has signs and symptoms of withdrawal if the drug intake is interrupted.

B. The phase of substance abuse when the substance abuse is long term and patterned.

C. A concentrated form of tetrahydrocannabinol made from boiling hashish.

D. The phase of substance abuse when the drug is used to help the individual accomplish a particular task.

E. Excessive use of mind or mood altering substances.

F. The phase of substance abuse when drugs are used at social gatherings.

G. An illness characterized by compulsion, loss of control, and continued patterns of abuse perceived negative consequences.

H. The phase of substance abuse when the abuse is short term and nonpatterned.

I. A potent concentrate of resin derived from the flowering tops of marijuana plants.

J. The last phase of substance abuse-addiction.

K. Substances that alter the normal functioning of the peripheral and central nervous systems.

L. The substance that alcohol is converted into in the liver.

STUDY QUESTIONS

13. Put the five phases of substance abuse in the correct order of occurrence.
    Circumstantial or situational, experimental, compulsive, intensified, social-recreational.

14. Contrast substance abuse with addiction.

15. Compare the three theories of substance abuse and addiction described in Chapter 12.

16. Name three physical manifestations of substance abuse for each body system.

    Central Nervous System:

    Immune System:

    Cardiovascular System:

    Gastrointestinal System:

    Reproductive System:

    Respiratory System:

17. List five cognitive and psychosocial manifestations of substance abuse.

COMPLETION EXERCISES

CENTRAL NERVOUS SYSTEM DEPRESSANT PROTOTYPE

ETHANOL

Description: Available in many different forms. One of the most common, frequently used drugs.

Pharmacokinetics: Rapidly absorbed from the (18.)_____ and (19.)_____.

Ingestion of (20.)_____ or _____ slows absorption of alcohol. Complete absorption takes (21.)_____ to _____ hours. After absorption, alcohol is distributed throughout the body. Most ingested alcohol is metabolized in the (22.)_____.

Pharmacodynamics: Exact mechanism of action is unclear. Possible explanations: with (23.)_____ constituents of brain cell membranes; increased blood levels of (24.)_____; interaction with the major (25.)_____ transmitter of the brain; effect on the amino acid that is the main (26.)_____ neurotransmitter of the brain.

Physiologic effects: Depresses the (27.)_____.

Undesired clinical responses: Affects almost every organ system of the body. Is converted to (28.)_____ in the liver, which is highly toxic to all organs.

Pharmacologic agent used to treat abuse: Disulfiram or (29.)_____ is analdehyde dehydrogenase inhibitor that raises the plasma level of (30.)_____ after alcohol ingestion, causing unpleasant reactions and decreasing the pleasure from ethanol.

CENTRAL NERVOUS SYSTEM STIMULANT PROTOTYPE

COCAINE

Description: Alkaloid from plant leaves.   White crystalline (31.)_____.
Dramatic increase in use. Preferred method is (32.)_____ or _____ for absorption through the nasal mucosa. Self-administered by other routes such as buccal membranes and intravenously.

Pharmacokinetics: Absorbed rapidly into bloodstream through nasal mucosa or buccal membranes. Very (33.)_____ half-life. Rapidly metabolized to benzoylecgonine by the (34.)_____. To maintain CNS stimulation must be inhaled or injected every (35.)_____ to _____ minutes.

Pharmacodynamics: Direct effects on (36.) _____ cells and alteration of central (37.) _____ levels. Inhibits reuptake of (38.) _____ at adrenergic synapses.

Undesired clinical responses: Intravenous injecting or smoking can cause sudden death as a result of ventricular (39.) _____ , myocardial infarction, cerebrovascular accident, or (40.) _____ arrest. Other cardiac, respiratory, and circulatory problems may occur, as well as (41.) _____ psychomotor reflexes and agitation and damage to the nasal septum.

Pharmacologic agents used to treat cocaine abuse: Antidepressants used to treat depression after discontinuing cocaine use. Desipramine hydrochloride (Norpramin, Pertofrane) is a tricyclic antidepressant that restores normal levels of (42.) _____ in the CNS.

Bromocriptine mesylate (Parlodel) and amantadine hydrochloride (Summetrel) are dopamine receptor agonists that suppress (43.) _____ and craving.

HALLUCINOGEN PROTOTYPE

MARIJUANA

Description: Psychoactive substance containing more than 400 chemicals. Primary psychoactive substance is (44.) _____ (THC), a concentrate in resin in (45.) _____ and leaves of marijuana plants. Potency depends on amount and potency of (46.) _____ . Available mostly as (47.) _____ —dried leaves, stems, and flowers of plant which are smoked or eaten in food. Also available as (48.) _____ , a potent resin concentrate, or hash oil, a very concentrated form of (49.) _____ .

Pharmacokinetics: Ingested marijuana is metabolized in the (50.) _____ . Inhaled marijuana is metabolized partly in the (51.) _____ . THC absorbed into circulation leaves the bloodstream rapidly. Stored in body compartments, highest concentration in (52.) _____ . THC slowly released back into systemic circulation. THC (53.) _____ are eliminated through feces and small amounts through urine. Detectable for up to 6 days after use.

Pharmacodynamics: Mechanisms of action not well understood. Affects brain amine levels, produces ultrastructural changes in some (54.) _____ and crosses biologic membranes.

Undesired clinical responses: Direct effects on (55.) _____ system. Also affects CNS, cardiovascular system, and (56.) _____ system.

CRITICAL THINKING ACTIVITY

Case Study: You are a nurse caring for a 24-year-old construction worker who has extensive orthopedic injuries from a fall at work. While you are in the room giving him medication for pain, he tells you he fell from the scaffolding because he was "high." Develop 5 questions you could use to assess him for substance abuse.

CHAPTER 13
DRUG THERAPY IN CHILDBEARING AND BREASTFEEDING CLIENTS

DEFINITION OF TERMS

Unscramble the term that fits the definition.

1. A drug that causes permanent alteration in form or function in a fetus. (geatrtneo)

   _____

2. The secretion and ejection of milk by the mammary glands. (tonalicat) _____

3. The part of the alveoli of the breast that produces breast milk. (lailehtipeoym leslc)

   _____ _____

4. The second to eighth week of pregnancy. (iormcnybe iporde) _____ _____

5. The substance produced by the breast for the first 3 to 4 days after birth. (roctusoml)

   _____

6. The hormone from the anterior pituitary gland that promotes lactation. (rapicolnt)

   _____

7. The growth in number and differentiation of cells to form organs and tissues. (nisogegosaren)

   _____

8. The period of pregnancy lasting from the eighth week to birth. (falet diproe) _____

   _____

9. The hormone released as a result of stimulation from infant sucking that prompts the myoepithelial cells to contract, compressing the alveoli and ejecting milk. (conxitoy)

   _____

10. The period of pregnancy from fertilization of the egg to the implantation of the products of conception into the uterus. (mouv) _____

11. The development of specialized cells to form organs and tissues. (lecl nitonifedaferit) _____

   _____

STUDY QUESTIONS

12. Identify five factors that affect placental transport of drugs.

13. Describe placental changes occurring late in gestation that increase the transfer of drugs.

14. Describe the affects of drugs on the fetus.

15. List 3 causes of low birth weight infants.

16. List 3 abnormalities of Fetal Alcohol Syndrome.

17. List 5 problems of neonates associated with cocaine use during pregnancy.

18. List 5 factors that influence the amount of drugs available in breast milk.

19. Why is it so important to assess drug use in pregnant and breast-feeding women?

20. Why are over-the-counter drugs a special concern for pregnant and breast-feeding women?

21. List one resource for determining if a particular drug is safe during pregnancy or breast-feeding.

MULTIPLE CHOICE

Select the best answer.

22. What types of drugs pass most easily into breast milk?
  A. drugs with large drug molecules
  B. drugs bound to plasma proteins
  C. lipid-soluble drugs
  D. ionized drugs

23. Which statement is most accurate about physiologic factors that influence drug absorption in the gastrointestinal system of newborns?
  A. Functional readiness of the GI tract involves gastric acid secretion and gastric emptying.
  B. Functional readiness of the GI tract depends on peristalsis, which become regular at 2 to 3 months of age.
  C. Gastric acid secretion, which is affected by type of delivery, is stable by 2 weeks of age.
  D. Breast fed infants have slower gastric emptying time.

24. Which answer is correct about physiologic factors that influence the distribution of drugs in newborns?
  A. Body fat content is higher in newborns; this produces slower release of drugs into the circulation.
  B. Protein binding is higher in newborns, leading to more free unbound drugs being available.
  C. Newborns have a greater total water content, which increases drug concentration.
  D. Newborns have a greater ratio of extracellular to intracellular fluid volume, decreasing extracellular drug concentration.

25. Which sentence best describes the physiologic influence on biotransformation in newborns?
  A. The infant's liver begins detoxifying at birth.
  B. The liver is the only organ that is capable of biotransformation.
  C. Hepatic enzymes are reduced during the neonatal period.
  D. Oxidation enzymes are the only hepatic enzymes that continue at fetal levels after birth.

26. Which one of the following most accurately describes the physiologic factor that influences renal excretion of drugs in newborns?
    A. Renal blood flow is influenced by the capacity of the glomerulus.
    B. The rate of glomerular filtration influences the rate of excretion of drugs.
    C. The glomerular filtration rate is the slowest kidney function to develop.
    D. Tubular secretion function usually reaches adult levels by 3 months of age.

CRITICAL THINKING ACTIVITIES

The nurse assesses a 17-year-old pregnant client. The client indicates that she uses cocaine occasionally even though she knows that she shouldn't. What action should be taken by the nurse?

CHAPTER 14
DRUG THERAPY IN THE NEONATE AND PEDIATRIC CLIENT

DEFINITION OF TERMS

Fill in the blanks.

An adolescent is a child between the onset of (1.)_____ and the cessation of (2.)_____ (approximately age (3.)_____ to (4.)_____).

An infant is a child from the end of the (5.)_____ of life to the end of the (6.)_____ of life.

A neonate is a (7.)_____.

A newborn is a child from the time of (8.)_____ through the (9.)_____ _____ of life.

A preschooler is a child between (10.)_____ and (11.)_____ years of age.

A school-age child is a child between (12.)_____ years of age and (13.)_____.

PLANNING AND IMPLEMENTING NURSING CARE

List one nursing measure that is developmentally appropriate when administering drugs for each age child.

14. Infants _____

15. Toddlers _____

16. Preschoolers _____

17. School age _____

18. Adolescence _____

PHARMACOKINETIC DIFFERENCES IN NEONATES, INFANTS, AND YOUNG CHILDREN

Complete the following:

ABSORPTION

Oral

Physiologic Factors   Results

19. Altered gastric pH less acidic in neonates &   _____
      under 3 years
                                                         _____

                                                         _____

                                                         Drugs remain in the stomach longer = more
20. _____   complete absorption of some drugs.
                                                         Acceleration of peak serum concentration = over
      _____   dose or toxicity

                                                         Drugs absorbed in the small intestine have re-
                                                         duced absorption = delay of peak serum concen-
                                                         tration level

21. Diminished enzymatic activities of small in-   _____
      testines
                                                         Decreased absorption of lipid-soluble drugs
22. Neonates: _____
and _____

Topical

23. Neonates and infants: _____
Proportionally more skin, thin skin, high water
  content, and increased vascularization

24. _____
                                                         Possibility of toxic affects

Parenteral

25. Neonates, infants, and young children: _____

Lower muscle mass
Body fat composition varies with age:
    highest in 1 year and 10-11 year olds
    lowest in preschoolers

MULTIPLE CHOICE

Select the best answer.

26. Which statement is most accurate about calculation of pediatric drug dosages?
    A. Clark's rule bases doses on the child's age and uses a nomogram to determine body surface area.
    B. Fried's and Young's rule base the dose on milligrams of drug per pounds of weight.
    C. Dose calculation according to body weight is the most accurate method, because it takes into account differences in maturational development.
    D. Dose calculation by body surface area is the most accurate method because it takes differences in size into account.

27. Which choice is most appropriate about administration of oral drugs to pediatric clients ?
    A. The nurse should collect the medicine from the infant "drool" and readminister to that infant.
    B. Honey is a good liquid to use for crushed tablets for infants because the honey tends to hold all of the particles together rather than leaving a residue.
    C. Measurement by teaspoons is just as accurate as the same amount in milliliters.
    D. If a drug is not supplied in liquid form, the nurse can always crush the tablet or use the capsule content in a liquid.

28. Which answer is correct about parenteral drug administration for pediatric clients?
    A. The recommended sites for intramuscular injections for children birth to 2 years of age are the gluteus maximus and dorsogluteal muscles.
    B. The recommended needle size for all children receiving injections is the 25 gauge needle.
    C. The vastus lateralis is the preferred intramuscular injection site for most age groups.
    D. The recommended site for subcutaneous injections for children is in the deltoid muscle.

29. Which sentence best describes drug efficacy and toxicity in pediatric clients?
    A. Dosage requirements of drugs for infants and children with disease states has been carefully studied by researchers.
    B. Drug efficacy is altered by disease states in infants and children.
    C. Children always require smaller doses of drugs than adults.
    D. All drugs are more toxic to infants than adults.

CHAPTER 15
DRUG THERAPY IN THE ELDERLY CLIENT

DEFINITION OF TERMS

In the columns of letters on the following page, find the words that complete the following statements. The hidden words run forward, backward, up, down, and diagonally.

1. Use of multiple drugs concurrently is called _____.

2. The term _____ is used to describe individuals 60 to 85 years old.

3. Individuals over the age of 85 years are called _____ _____.

4. _____ is the term used to describe biologic aging.

5. The study and treatment of diseases of the elderly is _____ .

6. The term _____ describes a visual change commonly seen in the elderly

7. The elderly may have impaired hearing or _____.

N	B	X	P	Z	H	D	V	S	G	P	C
T	M	I	T	E	L	D	E	R	L	Y	S
A	G	Q	R	V	N	O	R	M	A	L	E
I	X	E	K	E	L	L	Y	N	P	P	N
P	D	T	R	A	V	J	E	O	I	A	E
O	C	M	F	I	X	Y	L	D	N	H	S
Y	T	H	O	M	A	S	D	J	N	K	C
B	R	E	W	J	Q	T	E	U	E	L	E
S	T	Y	U	A	I	O	R	A	L	S	N
E	K	J	H	C	G	F	L	I	L	D	C
R	L	M	N	O	B	V	Y	X	C	Z	E
P	R	E	S	B	Y	C	U	S	I	S	T
Y	C	A	M	R	A	H	P	Y	L	O	P

On the figure below, indicate common physiologic changes associated with aging.

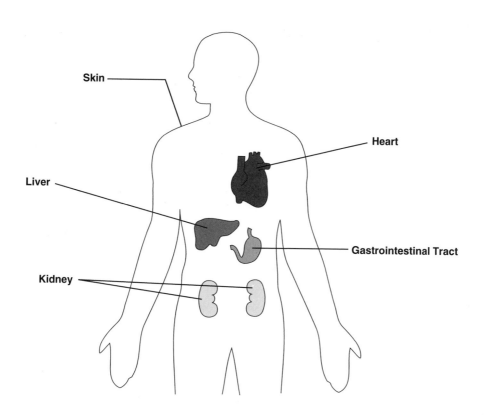

STUDY QUESTIONS

8. Describe how the following age-related changes affect drug absorption.
   Reduced perfusion and acidity of the GI tract:

   Reduced intestinal motility:

9. Compare the rate and quality of drug absorption in the elderly to drug absorption in the newborn

10. List four age-related changes that hinder drug distribution in the elderly. Explain the affect of each change.

11. Explain why the elderly client has an increased risk for adverse reactions.

MULTIPLE CHOICE

Select the correct answer.

12. Which one of the following represents a normal physiologic change associated with aging?
    A. lean body mass tends to decrease
    B. subcutaneous tissue tends to increase
    C. total body water in the elderly usually increases
    D. muscle mass proportionally increases

13. Which one of the following represents the effect of aging on cardiovascular function?
    A. increased cardiac output
    B. reduced arterial wall elasticity
    C. increased renal perfusion
    D. reduced peripheral vascular resistance

14. In the elderly, fat-soluble drugs are:
    A. distributed to a smaller portion of tissue than in young adults.
    B. absorbed at a slow rate due to reduced fat stores.
    C. released into circulation quickly after being absorbed.
    D. associated with increased duration of drug action.

15. The effect of aging on hepatic function results in:
    A. reduced plasma levels of drugs.
    B. prolonged drug effect.
    C. reduced incidence of toxicity.
    D. decreased intensity of drug effect.

CRITICAL THINKING ACTIVITY

There are many changes in metabolism and organ function in the elderly. These changes affect the pharmaceutic, pharmacodynamic, pharmacokinetic, and pharmacotherapeutic phases of drug therapy. Identify five essential drug-related interventions for the elderly client in the hospital. For the elderly client in the home?

Chapter 16
NURSE'S ROLE IN DRUG THERAPY IN THE HOME

Definition of Terms

Define the following.

1. Compliance

2. Interdisciplinary collaboration

3. Noncompliance

4. Priorities

Case Study

Charles Dickers is an 86 year old home health client with diagnoses of angina, arteriosclerotic heart disease, and cerebrovascular accident. His medications are digoxin 0.125 mg o.d.; enalapril 25 mg b.i.d.; Lasix 40 mg b.i.d.; isosorbide dinitrate 20 mg t.i.d.; and Coumadin 5 mg o.d.

Mr. Dickers is a widower who lives alone on a farm 20 minutes from a small town and several hours from the nearest city. He has been followed by a home health agency since a hospitalization one month ago for a mild cerebrovascular accident. His home health visits are covered by Medicare. He expresses a strong desire to remain independent in his own home.

On this visit, the nurse notes the usual clutter in his house, including unwashed dishes. Mr. Dickers finds his medications under some newspapers on the floor of the living room. He says that he just can't always remember to take his medicines and sometimes gets the bottles mixed up. The nurse's count of Coumadin shows that he has more tablets left and fewer Lasix tablets left than he should.

The nurse is drawing a blood specimen for a prothrombin time and digitalis level today.

The physical assessment shows a blood pressure of 130/80, pulse 52 and regular, and 2+ pitting edema of the ankles. He has no signs of irregular bleeding and his lungs are clear. Mr. Dickers appears depressed and says he "just doesn't care anymore" because he misses his wife so much.

5. Complete the "Home Medication Checklist" on p.136 of Chapter 16 for Mr. Dickers with the available information in the case study. From the information in the case study, you should have an idea on some of the areas of the checklist that are not specifically covered in the case study.

6. Based on your assessment, develop a nursing care plan to address Mr. Dickers problems.

Develop at least two nursing diagnoses and at least two expected outcomes for each diagnoses. Develop interventions for each nursing diagnosis.

Nursing diagnosis: Expected outcomes: Nursing diagnosis: Expected Outcomes:	Interventions

STUDY QUESTIONS

List potential problems for the following modalities of parenteral drug therapy used in home care.

7. Peripheral intravenous infusion: _____

_____

8. Central venous access: _____

_____

9. Ambulatory infusion pumps: _____

_____

10. What are the major concerns when using chemotherapy in the home? _____

_____

_____

CRITICAL THINKING ACTIVITY

What skills are especially important for the community health nurse in the management of drug therapy in the home?

Chapter 17
OVERVIEW OF THE CENTRAL NERVOUS SYSTEM

Definition of Terms

Complete the sentences, choosing the correct term for each definition.

Neuroglia, neuron, action potential, depolarization, neurotransmitter, polarization, resting potential, synapse, threshold potential.

1. The difference in electric charge between the sodium ions outside the neuron cell membrane and a greater concentration of potassium ions inside the cell membrane is _____ _____.

2. A cell of the central nervous system that supplies nutrients to the neuron, helps maintain the electric potential of the neuron, and phagocytizes waste products from injured neurons is a _____.

3. A chemical substance secreted by the presynaptic neuron into the synaptic cleft that acts on the receptor proteins in the membrane of the postsynaptic neuron to excite, inhibit, or modify its sensitivity is a _____.

4. The state of a neuron cell membrane when there is a positive charge on the outer surface and a negative charge on the inner surface is _____.

5. The state when a neuron cell membrane depolarizes and repolarizes is called _____.

6. The junction between the processes of neurons or between a neuron and an effector organ is a

    _____ .

7. The point at which the neuron cell membrane permeability changes to allow sodium ions to rush

    into the cell and potassium ions to diffuse outward is _____

    _____ .

8. A cell that conducts impulses in the central nervous system is a _____

9. The state when a neuron cell membrane loses its electric charge is _____

    _____ .

NEURON STRUCTURE AND FUNCTION

10-13. Write the name of each part of the neuron in the appropriate blank. Under each name, list the major function of that part of the neuron.

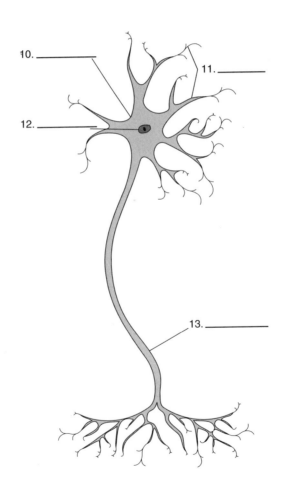

FUNCTIONS OF THE CNS STRUCTURES

Match the structures of the CNS with their functions or descriptions.

4. _____ Afferent division

5. _____ Basal ganglia

6. _____ Brain stem

7. _____ Cerebellum

8. _____ Cerebral cortex

9. _____ Cerebral hemispheres

10. _____ Cerebrum

11. _____ Diencephalon

12. _____ Efferent division

13. _____ Hypothalamus

14. _____ Limbic system

15. _____ Reticular formation

16. _____ Reticular activating system

17. _____ Thalamus

18. _____ Frontal lobe

19. _____ Parietal lobe

20. _____ Temporal lobe

31. _____ Occipital lobe

32. _____ Spinal cord

A. Contains the thalamus and hypothalamus

B. Carries action potentials away from the CNS

C. The lobe that controls interpretation of sensations, memory, behavior, emotion, and personality

D. The part of the brain stem that serves as a central relay system for sensory impulses ascending from other parts of the nervous system to the cerebral cortex

E. The lobe that controls motor activity, including speech, emotional expression, behavior, and abstract reasoning

F. Coordinates and refines muscle activity, and is important for equilibrium and proprioception

G. Transmits action potentials to the CNS

H. Receives input from higher brain regions that control skeletal muscles. Also influences auditory sense, equilibrium, and pain sensation

I. Serves as relay stations for motor impulses originating in the cerebral cortex and passing into the brain stem and spinal cord.

J. Conducts nerve impulses between brain and body parts

K. The lobe that controls processing sensory input, recognizing spatial relationships, and comprehending written communication

L. Connects the cerebrum to the spinal cord

M. Contain the major lobes

N. Plays a key role in maintaining homeostasis by regulating visceral activities and linking the nervous and endocrine systems

O. Alerts the cortex to incoming sensory signals, maintains consciousness and awakening from sleep

P. Contains nearly 75% of all the neurons in the nervous system

Q. The lobe that controls visual cortex and visual associative areas

R. Plays an important role in emotional responses

S. The largest part of the brain

MULTIPLE CHOICE

Select the best answer.

33. Which statement is most accurate about selective and nonselective drugs?

    A. Most drugs exhibit nonselective actions.
    B. Drugs with nonselective actions modify neurotransmitters.
    C. Drugs with specific actions increase the amount of the neurotransmitter at the synapse.
    D. Drugs with selective actions decrease the physiologic response to the neurotransmitter.

34. Which is the best example of a drugs with nonspecific actions?

    A. Anesthetic gases
    B. Anticonvulsants
    C. Antiemetics
    D. Antidepressants

35. Which answer is correct about the effect of drugs on the CNS?

    A. Drugs that act selectively to modify CNS function always depress neuron function.
    B. Drugs that act selectively produce effects on only one part of the CNS.
    C. CNS nonselective stimulants excite the CNS by increasing synaptic recovery time.
    D. CNS nonspecific depressants act by decreasing the amount of neurotransmitter release.

CRITICAL THINKING ACTIVITY

For each of the protective structures of the brain and spinal cord listed below, describe the protective mechanism and how this protection could become ineffective.

Example: 1. Bones of cranium and vertebrae: Protect the soft tissues of the brain and spinal cord from injury and penetration with a tough shell. Severe trauma could break this shell and injure or destroy tissue. For example, a penetrating injury to the cranium could push parts of the cranium inward and injure brain tissue.

Meninges:

Cerebrospinal fluid:

Blood-brain barrier:

CHAPTER 18
SEDATIVES, HYPNOTICS, AND ANXIOLYTICS

DEFINITION OF TERMS

Differentiate among the following:

anxiolytic drugs

hypnotic drugs

sedative drugs

BARBITURATES

Complete the following for the barbiturate prototype, phenobarbital.

Pharmacokinetics for Oral Dose

1. Onset of action occurs in approximately _____ _____.

2. Peak action occurs in _____ to _____ _____.

3. Duration of action is _____ to _____ _____.

4. Phenobarbital is metabolized in the _____.

5. The drug's half-life in adults is _____ to _____ _____.

6. Phenobarbital is excreted by the _____; _____ to _____ % of the drug is eliminated unchanged in the urine.

BENZODIAZEPINES

Complete the following for the benzodiazepine prototype, diazepam.

Pharmacokinetics for Oral Dose

7. Diazepam is _____ to _____ % protein bound.

8. The drug is _____ lipid soluble.

9. Generally, onset of action is _____ to _____ _____; action diminishes in _____ to _____ hours.

10. Peak action for diazepam occurs in _____ to _____ _____.

11. The half-life for diazepam is _____ to _____ _____.

The oldest group of sedative-hypnotics still used to treat anxiety and insomnia is the barbiturates. Match the barbiturate in Column A with the appropriate duration of action in Column B.

Column A		Column B	
12. _____	secobarbital (Seconal)	A.	ultra-short acting
13. _____	phenobarbital	B.	short-acting
14. _____	thiopental (Pentothal)	C.	long-acting

STUDY QUESTIONS

15. Explain what is meant by the statement: CNS depressants demonstrate cross-tolerance.

16. Explain what is meant by the statement: Diazepam's effects on the respiratory system is dose-related.

17. Discuss the effects of sedative, hypnotic, or anxiolytic drugs on the central nervous system.

18. What teaching should be given to a client being discharged on sedative, hypnotic, or anxiolytic drugs?

19. What is the effect of sedative, hypnotic, or anxiolytic drugs on the elderly?

20. List alternative measures for ensuring rest, relaxation, and sleep other than drugs.

21. You are the nurse scheduling administration times for diazepam. What pharma-cokinetic properties impact on your decision?

22. Explain the action of flumazenil, a benzodiazepine antagonist.

23. Provide rationale for the following interventions.

When administering phenobarbital, assess client carefully for drowsiness, depression, or lethargy.
Rationale:

Prepare parenteral solutions of phenobarbital and diazepam in separate syringes.
Rationale:

Anticipate that doses of Warfarin may be increased when administered concurrently with phenobarbital.
Rationale:

Check phenobarbital dosages for children and elderly clients carefully.

Rationale:

MULTIPLE CHOICE

Select the best answer.

24. Which one of the following statements best describes the physiologic action of barbiturates. Barbiturates:
    A. depress respirations.
    B. increase peristalsis.
    C. stimulate the central nervous system.
    D. increase gastric secretions.

25. Benzodiazepines, such as Valium, have which one of the following characteristics?
    A. metabolized by the kidneys
    B. not affected by other CNS depressants
    C. a high therapeutic index
    D. tolerated well by the elderly

26. Abrupt cessation of diazepam produces:
    A. respiratory depression and euphoria.
    B. mental confusion and cardiovascular stimulation.
    C. drowsiness and elevated blood pressure.
    D. anterograde amnesia and paradoxical agitation.

27. Which one of the following is correct regarding phenobarbital? Phenobarbital
    A. has the lowest lipid solubility of all barbiturates.
    B. is metabolized by the kidneys.
    C. is classified as a Controlled Substance Schedule III.
    D. is classified as a Pregnancy Category D drug.

28. Buspirone hydrochloride (BuSpar) is classified as:
    A. a barbiturate.
    B. an imidazopyridine.
    C. a benzodiazepine.
    D. an azapirone.

CRITICAL THINKING ACTIVITY

How does the knowledge that diazepam is highly lipid soluble impact on your care?

CHAPTER 19
OPIOID AND NONOPIOID ANALGESICS

DEFINITION OF TERMS

Match the term in Column A with the appropriate definition in Column B

Column A

1. _____ acute pain

2. _____ analgesic adjuvants

3. _____ analgesia

4. _____ chronic pain

5. _____ endorphin

6. _____ kappa receptor

7. _____ psychogenic

8. _____ mixed agonist antagonist

9. _____ neuromodulator

10. _____ somatogenic

11. _____ narcotic

12. _____ mu receptor

13. _____ opioid agonist

14. _____ opioid

15. _____ hyperanalgesia

16. _____ biochemical mediator

17. _____ sigma receptor

18. _____ nociceptor

19. _____ pain

20. _____ psychologic dependence

Column B

A. mechanical, chemical, or thermal receptors that perceive pain

B. originating in the body

C. addictive or habit-forming drug

D. increased sensitivity to stimulation that normally does not cause pain

E. absence of sensibility to pain

F. elements in the transmission of pain

G. receptors that mediate analgesia, respiratory depression, euphoria

H. bind to mu receptors to produce analgesia

I. refers to drugs that bind to opioid receptors

J. emotional or psychological origin

K. persistent pain

L. receptors that produce seizures, hallucinations, and increased irritability

M. unpleasant sensory and emotional experience

N. blocks opioid effect at mu receptor

O. protective mechanism; onset sudden

P. emotional reliance on drugs

Q. substance released when nociceptors are injured

R. nonanalgesic drugs effective against certain types of pain

S. neuropeptides that inhibit transmission of pain impulses

T. receptors that mediate analgesia, respiratory depression, miosis, and sedation

OPIOID ANALGESIC PROTOTYPE

Complete the following for morphine sulfate.

PHARMACOKINETICS

21. Onset of action occurs in approximately _____ _____ .

22. Peak action after IV bolus occurs in _____ to _____ _____ .

23. Duration of action after IM or SC is _____ to _____ _____ .

24. Morphine is metabolized in the _____ .

25. Morphine is excreted by the _____; _____ of the drug is found in the body after 48 hours.

PHARMACODYNAMICS

26. Morphine provides analgesia by binding to the _____ and _____ receptors.

OPIOID ANTAGONIST PROTOTYPE

Complete the following for naloxone.

PHARMACOKINETICS AND PHARMACODYNAMICS

27. Effects from an IM or SC injection of naloxone occurs within _____ to _____ _____ .

28. Naloxone is a _____ antagonist for _____, _____, _____, and _____ receptors.

STUDY QUESTIONS

29. What assessment data should you collect before administering an analgesic to the following clients? (Remember to use your growth and development background.)
    Five (5)-year-old child following a herniorrhaphy.

    Fourteen (14) year old with a fractured right femur.

    Fifty (50)-year-old aphasic male.

30. Compare pharmacodynamic properties of acetylsalicylic acid and acetaminophen.

31. All narcotic analgesics' potencies are compared to Morphine. How would the potency of the following drugs compare to Morphine 10 mg?
Codeine 60 mg; Levo-Dromoran 4 mg; Dilaudid 2 mg; Demerol 75 mg. (All drugs are for parenteral administration.)

32. Identify the signs and symptoms associated with the triad of opioid poisoning.

33. List three (3) mixed opioid agonist-antagonists. Explain the pharmacodynamics of each drug you listed.

MULTIPLE CHOICE

Select the best answer.

34. Morphine sulfate's effect on medullary centers includes stimulation of:
    A.   autonomic control over circulation.
    B.   cough reflex center.
    C.   chemoreceptor vomiting center.
    D.   respiratory rate and depth.

35. You are preparing to administer an injection of morphine to a client. You assess that the respiratory rate is 10 per minute. You should:
    A.   administer a smaller dose and record your findings.
    B.   notify the physician and delay drug administration.
    C.   administer the prescribed dose and notify the physician.
    D.   record your assessment data and assess again in 1 hour.

36. Drugs that contain or are extracted from opium are called:
    A.   opiates.
    B.   opioids.

37. Aspirin may be enteric coated:
    A.   to ensure dissolution in the small intestines instead of the stomach.
    B.   so that the dosage can be decreased.
    C.   to prevent decomposition of the drug.
    D.   to retard spoilage of the drug ingredients.

CRITICAL THINKING ACTIVITY

Read:

Fox, A.E. (1994). Ethical issues: Confronting the use of placebos for pain. *American Journal of Nursing*, 94(9), 42-45.

You are caring for a client scheduled to receive placebos for pain. The client asks you directly if the drug being administered is "fake." What ethical issues exist in this situation? How should you respond?

Hughes, T.L., & Smith. L. (1994). Is your colleague chemically dependent? *American Journal of Nursing*, 94(9), 30-35.

You suspect a colleague of substance abuse. What are the warning signs of chemical dependency? What actions should you take? What resources are available for nurses dependent on drugs?

Chapter 20
PSYCHOTHERAPEUTIC DRUGS

Definition of Terms

Define the following:

1. acute dystonia

2. akathisia

3. hypertensive crisis

4. irreversible inhibition

5. neuroleptic malignant syndrome

6. oculogyric crisis

7. poisthotonus

8. parkinsonism

9. reversible inhibition

10. tardive dyskinesia

LOW-POTENCY NEUROLEPTIC PROTOTYPE

Complete the following for chlorpromazine (Thorazine).

PHARMACOKINETICS

11.   Oral chlorpromazine is adsorbed _____ and _____ from the GI tract.

12.   Highest concentration of the drug occurs in the _____, _____, _____ _____, and _____.

13.   Chlorpromazine is _____ metabolized in the liver; clinical effects of a single dosage can last ___ hours.

PHARMACODYNAMICS

14.   Neuroleptic drugs block receptors for _____, _____, _____, and _____ .

MEDIUM-POTENCY NEUROLEPTIC PROTOTYPE

Complete the following for loxapine hydrochloride (Loxitane).

PHARMACOKINETICS

15.   Approximate half-life after an IM injection of loxapine is _____ to _____ hours.

HIGH-POTENCY NEUROLEPTIC PROTOTYPE

Complete the following for haloperidol (Haldol).

PHARMACOKINETICS

16.   Haloperidol peaks in _____ to _____ hours; duration of action is approximately _____ hours.

17.   The drug is _____ to _____ % plasma protein bound; half life is _____ to _____ hours.

STUDY QUESTIONS

18.   List and describe each of the major neurotransmitters involved in behavioral disorders.

19. Describe the four major groups of psychotherapeutic drugs.

20. Orthostatic hypotension may accompany the use of chlorpromazine. What instructions should be given to the client regarding how to diminish the effects of this condition?

21. Explain how aging impacts on plasma-protein binding of chlorpromazine.

22. Why is clozapine considered an atypical neuroleptic drug?

23. What instructions should be given the client regarding the anticholinergic side effects of neuroleptic drugs?

24. Distinguish between tertiary and secondary amine tricyclic antidepressants. Provide examples of each subtype.

25. Provide rationale for the following interventions.
    Asian clients must be assessed carefully for possible toxic levels of imipramine hydrochloride.
    Rationale:

Clients receiving tricyclic antidepressants must be carefully assessed for cardiovascular changes
Rationale:

Second-generation antidepressants are currently prescribed more frequently than first-generation drugs.
Rationale:

26. Describe the pharmacodynamics for each of the following antidepressant drugs.

imipramine hydrochloride

amitriptyline

nortriptyline

desipramine hydrochloride

fluoxetine

27. Lithium is effective against what disorders? Describe pharmacodynamic and pharmacotherapeutic properties of lithium.

28. Describe the use of drugs to treat major anxiety disorders.

MULTIPLE CHOICE

Select the best answer.

29. Antipsychotic drugs such as Thorazine (chlorpromazine) and Compazine (prochlorperazine) may also be used as:
    A.   analgesics.
    B.   antidepressants.
    C.   antiemetics.
    D.   analgesic antagonists.

30. During the maintenance phase of therapy with psychotherapeutic drugs:
    A.   the drug dosage is slowly reduced to a minimum dose.
    B.   the client's symptoms are ideally eliminated or reduced.
    C.   the drug dose is titrated upward to control symptoms.
    D.   the drug dosage is titrated downward to control symptoms.

31. Which one of the following is an anticholin-
ergic response associated with neuroleptic
drugs?
A.   blood dyscrasias
B.   lowered seizure threshold
C.   weight gain
D.   dry mouth

32. Anticholinergic blockade by antidepressant
drugs can produce which one of the follow-
ing:
A.   reflex tachycardia.
B.   tremors.
C.   constipation.
D.   erectile dysfunction.

33. Which one of the following statements ac-
curately describes the action of fluoxetine
hydrochloride? Fluoxetine hydrochloride
(Prozac):
A.   inhibits neuronal uptake of serotonin.
B.   acts as a histamine blocker.
C.   blocks the reuptake of norepinephrine.
D.   acts as an alpha-adrenergic blocker.

CRITICAL THINKING ACTIVITY

Before administering phenelzine (an MAO inhibitor) to a client, you collect a nutritional history. Why are you concerned with the client's dietary intake? What food
items are specifically a concern? What problem may develop if the client consumes
these food items while receiving phenelzine?

CHAPTER 21
ANTIEPILEPTIC DRUGS

DEFINITION OF TERMS

Match the terms in Column A with the appropriate definition in Column B. Use each answer only once.

Column A		Column B
1. ____ atonic	A.	rigid, violent muscular contractions; loss of consciousness
2. ____ absence		
3. ____ clonic	B.	brief, single, mild-to-moderate jerks of arms or head
4. ____ myoclonic	C.	sudden loss of muscle tone, leading to head drop or slumping of body
5. ____ tonic	D.	sudden, brief impairment of consciousness
6. ____ tonic-clonic	E.	generalized rigid, violent muscular contractions followed by rhythmic contractions and loss of consciousness
	F.	rhythmic, multiple jerks of all body parts with loss of consciousness

HYDANTOINS PROTOTYPE

Complete the following for phenytoin (Dilantin).

Pharmacokinetics

7. Most oral phenytoin absorption occurs in the _____ _____.
8. The drug is almost _____% plasma protein bound in adults.
9. After an oral dose, peak blood level is reached in approximately _____ to _____ hours. The average half-life of phenytoin is _____ hours.
10. Phenytoin is _____ metabolized in the liver.

Pharmacodynamics

11. Phenytoin acts mainly in the _____ _____ to normalize abnormal fluxes of _____ across neuron cell membranes.
12. Plasma concentrations from _____ to _____ μg/ml are therapeutically effective.

SUCCINIMIDE PROTOTYPE

Complete the following for ethosuximide (Zarontin).

Pharmacokinetics

13. Approximate half-life after an oral dose of ethosuximide is _____ hours in children and _____ hours in adults.

14. Most of the drug is metabolized in the liver and excreted in the urine. Approximately _____ to _____ % is excreted unchanged; approximately _____ to _____ % is excreted as an inactive derivative.

OXAZOLIDINEDIONE PROTOTYPE

Complete the following for trimethadione (Tridione).

Pharmacokinetics

15. Trimethadione peaks in _____ to _____ minutes; elimination half-life is _____ to _____ days.

16. Therapeutic levels of the drug may not be reached for more than _____ days.

STUDY QUESTIONS

17. Describe common drug-nutrient interactions associated with phenytoin therapy. What is the role of the nurse in regard to these interactions?

18. What instructions regarding oral hygiene should be given to the client receiving phenytoin?

19. What types of seizures respond to phenobarbital therapy? Describe the pharmacodynamic properties of phenobarbital that produce its effectiveness as an antiepileptic drug.

20. Primidone (Myidone, Mysoline) is nearly identical in structure to what other antiepileptic drug?

21. Therapeutic levels of trimethadione may not be reached for more than 30 days. What impact does this information have on the nursing care of the client receiving the drug?

22. Provide rationale for the following interventions.

Review results of baseline CBC and liver function studies before administering initial dose of carbamazepine.
Rationale:

Instruct the client to take carbamazepine with meals.
Rationale:

Assess the client receiving carbamazepine for bruising, sore throat, fever, petechiae, and mouth ulcerations.
Rationale:

23. Describe the pharmacodynamics for each of the following antidepressant drugs.

valproic acid

felbamate

diazepam

MULTIPLE CHOICE

Select the best answer.

24. The client receiving phenobarbital for seizures would be observed for which one of the following undesired responses?
    A. tachycardia
    B. blurred vision
    C. polyuria
    D. drowsiness

25. Most antiepileptic drugs act by:
    A. inhibiting the vasomotor center in the brain.
    B. suppressing sinoatrial node activity.
    C. depressing nerve cell excitability.
    D. facilitating peripheral muscle function.

26. The client receiving phenytoin reports to the nurse that she has started to use birth control pills. The teaching plan for this client should include information about the:
    A. hazards of pregnancy for women with seizures.
    B. risk for increased seizure activities.
    C. potential for decreased effectiveness of birth control pills while taking phenytoin.
    D. risk of thrombophlebitis while taking phenytoin and birth control pills.

CRITICAL THINKING ACTIVITY

Your client is taking antiepileptic drugs; increasing seizure activity suggests lack of drug effectiveness. What information should you collect from the client? Why would you recommend monitoring plasma drug levels?

CHAPTER 22
CENTRAL NERVOUS SYSTEM STIMULANTS

DEFINITION OF TERMS

Define the following:

1. amphetamine

2. attention deficit-hyperactivity disorder

3. caffeine

4. narcolepsy

5. nicotine

CEREBRAL STIMULANT: AMPHETAMINE

Complete the following for amphetamine sulfate.

Pharmacokinetics

6. Oral amphetamine sulfate is distributed into most body tissues, particularly the _____and _____ _____ _____.

7. Pharmacologic effects persist for _____ to _____ hours.

Pharmacodynamics

8. Amphetamine is a mixture of dextroamphetamine and levamphetamine. These two substances are _____, substances whose molecular structures are mirror opposites of each other.

Pharmaceutics

9. Amphetamine is administered exclusively by the _____ _____.

STUDY QUESTIONS

10. Discuss the rationale for amphetamine use in the treatment of attention deficit hyperactivity disorder.

11. Describe the physiologic effects of amphetamine on the following body systems:

    central nervous system

    respiratory system

    genitourinary system

12. List common undesired responses associated with amphetamine for the following body systems.

    central nervous system

    cardiovascular system

    gastrointestinal system

    Summarize appropriate nursing interventions associated with these effects.

13. Describe three clinical uses for caffeine.

14. Summarize the undesired effects of caffeine on the following body systems:

central nervous system

cardiovascular system

gastrointestinal system

urinary system

15. Describe the effects of chronic overuse of caffeine.

16. Nicotine is a ganglionic stimulating drug. Describe the physiologic responses to this drug.

17. Discuss the clinical indications for nicotine replacement therapy.

MULTIPLE CHOICE

Select the best answer.

18. Currently, the most widespread use of amphetamines is:
    A. for treatment of obesity.
    B. for treatment of asthma.
    C. as a respiratory stimulant.
    D. as a drug of abuse.

19. Which one of the following is the drug of choice for attention deficit hyperactivity disorder?
    A. amphetamine
    B. fenfluramine
    C. methylphenidate
    D. benzphetamine

20. Analeptics are used to:
    A. stop convulsions.
    B. promote gastrointestinal function.
    C. reduce laryngeal edema.
    D. stimulate respirations.

CRITICAL THINKING ACTIVITY

The parents of a child with ADHD questions the use of drugs for the treatment of their son's disorder. How would you answer their concerns?

Chapter 23
DRUGS USED TO TREAT PARKINSON'S DISEASE

Definition of Terms

Define the following:

1. akinesia

2. anhidrosis

3. bradykinesia

4. cogwheel rigidity

5. decarboxylation

6. extrapyramidal

7. idiopathic

8. Parkinsonian crisis

9. pyramidal

10. rest tremors

MULTIPLE CHOICE

Select the best answer.

1. Which statement is most accurate?
    A. Parkinson's disease is caused by the selective and progressive degeneration of the acetylcholine producing cells.
    B. The underlying cause of the progressive neuron cell degeneration in Parkinson's disease is unknown.
    C. Dopamine increases the production of acetylcholine, increasing the excitatory influence on the basal ganglia.
    D. The stimulation of basal ganglia by acetylcholine results in increased muscle tone in the body, allowing for refinement of voluntary movement.

2. What is currently known about the causes of Parkinson's disease?
    A. Most cases of Parkinson's disease are iatrogenic in origin.
    B. Postencephalitic parkinsonism symptoms can develop 30 years after the viral infection.
    C. Idiopathic Parkinson's disease is a common side effect of most antipsychotic drugs.
    D. Iatrogenic parkinsonism is believed to be caused by the loss of neurons with aging.

3. Which answer best describes the pharmacodynamics of drugs used to treat Parkinson's disease?
    A. The major goal of drug therapy is to enhance acetylcholine activity.
    B. The major goal of drug therapy is to regenerate dopamine-containing neurons.
    C. The major goal of drug therapy is to act as a dopamine antagonist.
    D. The major goal of drug therapy is to balance cholinergic and dopaminergic activity.

14. What should you tell a client receiving levodopa about drug-nutrient interactions?
    A. Levodopa should not be taken with meals because it slows absorption of the drug.
    B. A high protein diet should be consumed with this drug to enhance conversion of dopamine.
    C. Vitamin B_6 reverses the therapeutic effectiveness of levodopa.
    D. Consumption of high levels of pyridoxine with levodopa increases the duration action of levodopa.

15. Which choice best describes the drug-drug interaction of levodopa and carbidopa?
    A. Carbidopa decreases levodopa conversion in the periphery, increasing the levodopa going to the brain.
    B. Carbidopa increases the inhibitory effect of pyridoxine on levodopa, which results in a reduction of dosage of levodopa.
    C. Administering both drugs may delay the appearance of dosage-related reactions.
    D. Carbidopa crosses the blood-brain barrier to increase the metabolism of levodopa in the brain.

16. Which statement is most accurate about dopamine agonists?
    A. They are effective to alter the dyskinesia and on-off phenomenon associated with levodopa therapy.
    B. Their undesired clinical responses are completely different from levodopa therapy because they are ergot derivatives.
    C. They are much more potent than levodopa.
    D. They are useful for end-of-dose failure from long term use of levodopa.

DRUGS USED TO TREAT PARKINSON'S DISEASE

List an example of each type of drug.

Drugs to increase dopamine brain levels 17. _____

Decarboxylase inhibitors 18. _____

DRUGS —— Dopamine-releasing drugs 19. _____

Dopamine agonists   20. _____

Antimuscarinic or anticholinergic drugs 21. _____

DRUG PROTOTYPES

Fill in the blanks.

Description

Levodopa	Amantadine Hydrochloride
Increases dopamine brain levels. A (22) _____ that is the precursor to dopamine. Examples: L-dopa, Dopar, Larodopal	Releases dopamine. A synthetic antiviral agent Given with (23) _____ or anticholinergic therapy Examples: Symmetrel

Pharmacotherapeutics

Levodopa	Amantadine Hydrochloride
75% of patients improve. Rigidity and bradykinesia improve more than (24) _____. Improvement usually in 2nd or 3rd week of therapy, but sometimes not until 6 months. Therapeutic effectiveness declines after about 6 years. (25) _____ _____ phenomena	$^2/_3$ of patients improve, but not as effective as levodopa. Akinesia, rigidity, tremor, gait, and functional ability improve (26) _____ improvement (sometimes within 2 days) Optimal results in 3 months Short-term improvement developing (27) _____ in about 3 years.

Pharmacokinetics

Levodopa	Amantadine Hydrochloride
Absorbed from GI tract. Metabolized in GI tract and liver. Only 1% enters brain and is converted to (28) _____. 95% is converted to dopamine peripherally and (29) _____ be used by the CNS. Onset of action 30-45 minutes. Peak plasma concentrations 1-3 hours. Ingestion with food (30) _____ absorption. 80% excreted in urine within 24 hours.	Absorbed from (31) _____ _____. Peak blood concentrations in 1-4 hours. Elimination half-life averages 24 hours. Drug excreted unchanged in urine.

Pharmacodynamics

Levodopa	Amantadine Hydrochloride
It is a catecholamine that is the metabolic precursor of dopamine. Crosses blood-brain barrier (dopamine cannot). Effects thought to be related to newly formed (32) _____.	Exact mechanism of action (33) _____. Thought to act by releasing dopamine from dopaminergic terminals that have not degenerated.

Undesired Clinical Responses

Levodopa	Amantadine Hydrochloride
(34) _____ reactions that improve with tolerance to drug: anorexia, nausea, vomiting (35) _____ _____ Cardiac arrhythmias Drowsiness, fatigue Excitation, anxiety, insomnia Mydriasis Choreiform movements Late reactions increasing with duration of therapy: (36) _____ Dark-colored urine and perspiration Urinary retention or frequency Hemolytic anemia Mental (15%)= depression, vivid dreams, delusions, visual hallucinations	Mild CNS disturbances: Dizziness, insomnia, nervousness, anxiety, hallucinations, confusion, nightmares, and impaired ability to concentrate. (37)_____with adjustment of dosage. Appear within few hours of initiating therapy or changing drug dosage. Nausea Drowsiness, lethargy, and slurred speech (38) Livedo reticularis=reddish blue mottle discoloration of _____ and sometimes _____. Common, but not serious.

Contraindications and Precautions

Levodopa	Amantadine Hydrochloride
History of myocardial infarction with residual (39) _____. Sympathomimetic drugs for bronchial asthma or emphysema Severe cardiovascular, pulmonary, renal, hepatic, endocrine, or active peptic ulcer disease Wide-angle glaucoma (40)_____ disorders	(41) _____ disease Recurrent eczematoid dermatitis Uncontrolled psychosis (42) _____ CNS-stimulating drugs Impaired renal functioning (43) _____ _____ _____ Peripheral edema Orthostatic hypotension

Drug-Drug Interactions

Levodopa	Amantadine Hydrochloride
Numerous interactions Interacts with: Monoamine oxidase (MAO) inhibitors result in dopamine buildup which could cause (44) _____ _____ and hyperpyrexia. MAO inhibitor selegiline hydrochloride results in extending the duration of action of (45)_____. Phenothiazine and butyrophenone sedatives result in antagonism of the therapeutic effects of levodopa. (46) _____ , including tricyclic result in orthostatic hypotension.	Interacts with anticholinergic drugs resulting in (47) _____ clinical responses from the anticholinergic drugs.

Specific Nursing Considerations

Levodopa	Amantadine Hydrochloride
Causes elevated serum and urinary pH levels, false-positive reactions for urinary (48) _____ and ketones, false elevations of urinary catecholamine results. (49) _____ require lower doses. Monitor (50)_____ _____closely during initiation of adjustment of drug therapy. Safety when changing position because of (51) _____ _____. Observe for changes in personality or behavior Signs of overdose: muscle twitching and spasmodic winking	If insomnia develops, evening dose should be taken (52) _____ _____ _____ _____. Monitor respiratory status, fluid retention, and weight on clients with history of (53) _____ _____ _____. Safety measures because of (54) _____.

CRITICAL THINKING ACTIVITY

Antonia Adolph is a 67-year-old retired attorney who was diagnosed with Parkinson's disease recently by her physician in a University hospital clinic. Her physician prescribed L-dopa three times a day. You are the nurse responsible for teaching Antonia how to manage her disease. She has the following symptoms: bradykinesia, fatigue, dysphagia, tremors of the hands, and a shuffling gate. Antonia is very well groomed and attractive. She is very active in voluntary legal aid programs. She appears distraught and says she feels like her life is over.

Develop a nursing care plan for Antonia with three nursing diagnoses, expected outcomes, interventions, and methods of evaluating your plan.

Nursing diagnosis and expected outcomes	Interventions	Evaluation methods
1.		
2.		
3.		

CHAPTER 24
ANESTHETIC AGENTS

DEFINITION OF TERMS

Define the following:

1. autonomic activity

2. blood-gas partition coefficient

3. emergence phase

4. induction phase

5. maintenance phase

6. minimum alveolar concentration

7. somatic responses

Match the characteristics in Column A with the appropriate phase of general anesthesia in Column B. Answers in Column B are used more than one time.

	Column A		Column B
8. _____	amount of anesthetic is gradually reduced	A.	induction phase
		B.	maintenance phase
9. _____	lasts from skin incision to closure of surgical wound	C.	emergence phase
0. _____	autonomic activity, muscle and somatic reflexes are regained		
1. _____	rapid loss of consciousness		
2. _____	characterized by unconsciousness, analgesia, muscle relaxation, obtunded reflexes, and autonomic blockade		
3. _____	neuromuscular blocking agents may be administered		
4. _____	onset of analgesia		
5. _____	progressive loss of muscle tone and autonomic activity		

PREOPERATIVE NURSING CARE

Choose one sedative, one analgesic, and one antimuscarinic drug from the list on page 248 of Chapter 24. Describe pharmacodynamic properties of the drug and related nursing interventions.

Sedative:

Analgesic:

Antimuscarinic:

STUDY QUESTIONS

16. List four inhalation anesthetics currently in use.

17. Describe the pharmacodynamic properties of halothane. How do these properties impact on th postoperative care of the client?

18. Describe the pharmacokinetic and pharmacodynamic properties of thiopental, an ultrashort acting barbiturate. How do these properties impact on the postoperative care of the client?

19. Identify three nonbarbiturate drugs used for induction of general anesthesia.

20. Describe the pharmacokinetic and pharmacodynamic properties of ketamine, a nonbarbiturate

21. Describe the pharmacokinetic and pharmacodynamic properties of fentanyl, an opioid use during the induction and maintenance phases of anesthesia.

CRITICAL THINKING ACTIVITY

Explain the statement: All potent inhalation anesthetics produce a dose-related CNS depression.

CHAPTER 25
OVERVIEW OF THE AUTONOMIC NERVOUS SYSTEM

DEFINITION OF TERMS

Define the following:

1. acetylcholinesterase

2. acetylcholine

3. adrenergic

4. afferent

5. alpha receptors

6. autonomic tone

7. beta receptors

8. cholinergic

9. efferent

10. epinephrine

11. ganglia

12.   muscarinic receptors

13.   neurotransmitter substances

14.   nicotinic receptors

15.   norepinephrine

16.   postganglionic and preganglionic neurons

17.   postganglionic and preganglionic fibers

STUDY QUESTIONS

18.   Identify the anatomic terms used to describe the two parts of the autonomic division of the peripheral nervous system.

19.   Pre- or postganglionic fibers that release acetylcholine are called _____.

20.   Postganglionic fibers that release epinephrine are called _____.

21.   List the primary neurotransmitters of the autonomic nervous system.

22.   Describe the role of neurotransmitters and neuroreceptors of the ANS as a basis for neuropharmacologic intervention.

23.   Cite general differences of adrenergic and cholinergic responses upon effector tissues: heart, liver, muscle, sweat glands.

4. Describe how and in what circumstances epinephrine is delivered to effector tissues.

5. List the two types of adrenergic receptors and the associated response of effector tissues.

6. Describe general effects of drugs on the autonomic nervous system.

MULTIPLE CHOICE

Select the best answer.

7. The autonomic nervous system includes both cholinergic and adrenergic nerves. Which one of the following is classified as adrenergic?
   A.   preganglionic sympathetic
   B.   preganglionic parasympathetic
   C.   postganglionic sympathetic
   D.   postganglionic parasympathetic

28. Parasympathomimetic or cholinergic drugs:
    A.   act like mediators of the adrenal medulla.
    B.   block the action of the parasympathetic nervous system.
    C.   act like mediators of the parasympathetic nervous system.
    D.   block the action of the sympathetic nervous system.

CRITICAL THINKING ACTIVITY

The client becomes fearful before surgery. His pulse is 120; blood pressure is 176/94, and his skin is cool and clammy. Is this client experiencing mass or discrete stimulation of the sympathetic nervous system? Why did you make this choice?

The client is working in the yard and becomes very warm. Soon he is perspiring profusely. Is this client experiencing mass or discrete stimulation of the sympathetic nervous system? Why did you make this choice?

CHAPTER 26
DRUGS AFFECTING THE PARASYMPATHETIC NERVOUS SYSTEM

DEFINITION OF TERMS

Define the following:

1. anticholinergic

2. cholinergic crisis

3. chronotropic

4. cycloplegia

5. inotropic

6. miosis

7. myasthenia crisis

8. myopia

9. pseudocholinesterase

10. xerostomia

PHYSIOLOGIC RESPONSE OF ORGANS TO ANTIMUSCARINIC DRUGS

Indicate the term that best describes the body's physiologic response to antimuscarinic drugs. Use the terms: dilate, constrict, increase, decrease, contract, relax, or no effect.

1. Salivary glands   _____

2. Sweat glands   _____

3. Bronchial secretion   _____

4. Bronchial smooth muscle   _____

5. GI tract smooth muscle   _____

6. Biliary tract smooth muscle   _____

7. Urinary bladder smooth muscle   _____

8. Eye   _____

9. Lacrimal glands   _____

20. Arteries   _____

21. Exocrine glands   _____

Identify the major undesired clinical responses associated with antimuscarinic drugs

System	**Undesired Clinical Response**
22. Gastrointestinal	_____
23. Integumentary	_____
24. Respiratory	_____
25. Sensory	_____
26. Urinary	_____
27. Cardiovascular	_____
29. Male reproductive	_____

PHYSIOLOGIC RESPONSE OF ORGANS TO PARASYMPATHETIC DRUGS

Indicate the body's physiologic response to parasympathomimetic drugs.

30. Exocrine glands   _____

31. Lungs   _____

32. Eye   _____

33. Gastrointestinal tract   _____

34. Urinary tract   _____

35. Heart   _____

36. Veins   _____

37. Arteries   _____

STUDY QUESTIONS

38. Provide the rationale for the following nursing interventions.
     Offer ice chips or sugarless, hard candy to the client receiving atropine sulfate.
     Rationale:

     Teach client receiving benztropine, an antimuscarinic drug, to avoid prolonged exposure to warm environments.
     Rationale:

     Increase oral fluid intake and dietary fiber, if not contraindicated, for client receiving benztropine an antimuscarinic drug.
     Rationale:

39. What are the antidotes for antimuscarinic drug?

40. Why is atropine used as a preoperative agent?

41. Describe the Tensilon Test, including nursing considerations.

2. Describe important nursing interventions for the client receiving ganglionic blockers.

3. List the four main uses for parasympathomimetic drugs.

4. What over-the-counter drugs should be avoided by clients receiving parasympathomimetic drugs.

5. Compare and contrast direct-acting vs indirect-acting parasympathomimetic drugs.

6. Why are most acetylcholinesterase inhibitors ineffective in treating central nervous system symptoms associated with insufficient acetylcholine?

7. Why do high doses of anticholinesterase drugs produce muscle weakness?

8. What signs and symptoms would clients with agricultural insecticide poisoning display?

MULTIPLE CHOICE

Select the best answer.

49. Antimuscarinic drugs compete with which one of the following neurotransmitters?
    A.   dopamine
    B.   acetylcholine
    C.   epinephrine
    D.   norepinephrine

50. The major undesired response associated with ganglionic blockers is:
    A.   bradycardia
    B.   tachycardia
    C.   hypotension
    D.   hypertension

51. The presence of which condition would contraindicate the use of acetylcholinesterase?
    A.   hypothyroidism
    B.   Raynaud's disease
    C.   pheochromocytoma
    D.   diabetes mellitus

52. Which of the following categories of drugs are used as an antidote to organophosphate poisoning?
    A.   parasympathomimetic
    B.   anticholinergic
    C.   antimuscarinic
    D.   sympathomimetic

CRITICAL THINKING ACTIVITY

Why do arteries and veins respond to exogenous acetylcholine administration even though they are not innervated by the parasympathetic nervous system?

Why are anticholinesterase drugs more appropriate to use in clients with myasthenia gravis than parasympathomimetic agents?

Chapter 27
DRUGS AFFECTING THE SYMPATHETIC NERVOUS SYSTEM

Definition of Terms

Define the following:

1. analeptic effect

2. anorexigenic effect

3. sympatholytic

4. sympathomimetic

PHYSIOLOGIC RESPONSE OF TARGET ORGANS TO ALPHA STIMULATION

Indicate the term that best describes the body's physiologic response to alpha stimulation. Use the terms: dilate, constrict, increase, decrease, contract, relax, or no effect.

5. Bronchial glands   _____

6. GI tract motility   _____

7. GI tract sphincters   _____

8. Arterioles and large veins   _____

9. Pregnant uterus   _____

10. Eye (iris, dilator muscle)   _____

PHYSIOLOGIC RESPONSE OF TARGET ORGANS TO BETA STIMULATION

Indicate the term that best describes the body's physiologic response to beta stimulation. Use the terms: dilate, constrict, increase, decrease, contract, relax, or no effect.

11. Bronchial smooth muscles   _____

12. Insulin secretion   _____

13. Heart   _____

14. Arterioles and large veins   _____

15. Detrusor muscle   _____

16. Renin secretion   _____

SYMPATHETIC AGONISTS

Match the generic names of sympathetic agonists with the appropriate trade or brand name.

17. ____   epinephrine   A.   Vasoxyl

18. ____   isoproterenol hydrochloride   B.   Aldomet

19. ____   phenylephrine hydrochloride   C.   Proventil

20. ____   albuterol sulfate   D.   Isuprel

21. ____   methoxamine hydrochloride   E.   Vasodilan

                                            F.   Adrenalin

                                            G.   Neo-Synephrine

STUDY QUESTIONS

22. Provide the rationale for the following nursing interventions associated with parenteral sympathomimetic drug administration:
     Before administering, inspect the solution carefully.
     Rationale:

     Use large central veins for intravenous sites.
     Rationale:

     Routinely evaluate pulses distal to intravenous sites.
     Rationale:

Monitor the client's vital signs carefully and frequently.
Rationale:

Following IM or SQ administration of epinephrine, massage the injection site well.
Rationale:

23. What information should be included in the discharge teaching of a client receiving sympatho-mimetic drugs?

24. List the four categories of α-blockers and describe the pharmacodynamic properties for each category.

25. Provide the rationale for the following nursing interventions associated with sympatholytic drug administration:
Monitor the blood pressure and heart rate carefully.
Rationale:

Administer intravenous alpha blocker via an infusion pump.
Rationale:

Teach the client receiving an oral alpha blocker how to count their own pulse.
Rationale:

Monitor the client carefully for faintness or syncope.
Rationale:

MULTIPLE CHOICE

Select the best answer.

26. Most undesired responses associated with direct-acting sympathomimetic drugs result from:
    A.   bronchiole dilating actions.
    B.   vasoconstriction effects.
    C.   relaxation of smooth muscle.
    D.   diminished secretions of glands.

27. Which one of the following drugs should be discontinued at least 2 weeks prior to the administration of sympathomimetic drugs?
    A.   cardiac glycosides
    B.   ACE inhibitors
    C.   calcium channel blockers
    D.   MAO inhibitors

28. Intravenous sympathomimetic drugs should not be mixed in which one of the following solutions?
    A.   acidic solutions
    B.   hypertonic solutions
    C.   alkaline solutions
    D.   hypotonic solutions

29. The primary therapeutic use of alpha blockers is to treat:
    A.   hypotension.
    B.   hypertension.
    C.   migraine headaches.
    D.   urinary retention.

30. The primary therapeutic use of ergot alkaloids is to treat:
    A.   hypotension.
    B.   hypertension.
    C.   migraine headaches.
    D.   Raynaud's phenomenon.

31. The nurse teaches the client going home on an alpha blockers not to discontinue the drug abruptly because:
    A.   severe hypotension may occur.
    B.   future control of blood pressure will be impossible.
    C.   achieving appropriate blood levels will take twice as long.
    D.   rebound hypertension could result.

CRITICAL THINKING ACTIVITY

The client is scheduled to have several skin lesions removed. A local anesthetic of Xylocaine and epinephrine will be used. Why is epinephrine combined with the Xylocaine solution?

CHAPTER 28
SKELETAL MUSCLE RELAXANTS

DEFINITION OF TERMS

Define the following:

1. curare

2. depolarizing neuromuscular blocking drugs

3. nondepolarizing neuromuscular blocking drugs

4. peripherally acting skeletal muscle relaxants

NONDEPOLARIZING NEUROMUSCULAR BLOCKING PROTOTYPE

Complete the following for tubocurarine hydrochloride.

Pharmacotherapeutics

5. Tubocurarine is used _____

_____.

Pharmacokinetics

6. Onset of effects following a single intravenous dose of tubocurarine to an adult occurs within ___ minute(s); maximum paralysis of muscles occurs within _____ to _____ minutes, and duration of effective paralysis lasts _____ to _____ minutes.

Pharmacodynamics

7. Tubocurarine produces its effects by competing with _____ for _____ _____ sites on motor end-plates.

DEPOLARIZING NEUROMUSCULAR BLOCKING PROTOTYPE

Complete the following for succinylcholine.

Pharmacokinetics

8. After an IV injection, onset of action occurs in _____ seconds or less; maximum effects are achieved

    within _____ minute(s), and muscle function returns to normal within _____ to _____ minutes.

9. Succinylcholine is rapidly degraded by _____.

PERIPHERALLY ACTING SKELETAL MUSCLE RELAXANT PROTOTYPE

Complete the following for dantrolene (Dantrium).

Pharmacokinetics

10. Dantrolene peaks in approximately _____ hours after oral administration.

11. After IV infusion, the blood concentration level remains at a steady state for approximately _____

    hours.

12. The drug's plasma half-life is ___ hours in adults and ___ hours in children.

STUDY QUESTIONS

13. List common undesired clinical responses associated with the drug dantrolene.

14. Develop a plan of care for the client with the following nursing diagnosis: High risk for altered
    elimination (constipation) related to decreased intestinal peristalsis associated with some skeletal
    muscle relaxant therapy.

CRITICAL THINKING ACTIVITY

Provide the rationale for the following statement: recovery from tubocurarine neuro-muscular blockade can be hastened by the administration of a cholinesterase inhibitor.

Chapter 29
OVERVIEW OF THE CARDIOVASCULAR SYSTEM

Definition of Terms

Define the following:

1. afterload

2. automaticity

3. autoregulation

4. capacitance

5. conductivity

6. contractility

7. diastole

8. preload

9. rhythmicity

10. systole

ANATOMY OF THE CARDIOVASCULAR SYSTEM

Complete the following diagram on anatomic structures of the heart.

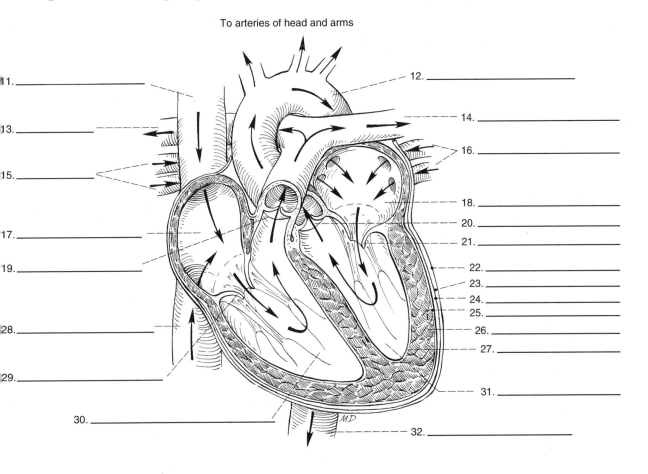

To arteries of head and arms

11. _____

13. _____

15. _____

17. _____

19. _____

28. _____

29. _____

30. _____

12. _____

14. _____

16. _____

18. _____

20. _____

21. _____

22. _____

23. _____

24. _____

25. _____

26. _____

27. _____

31. _____

32. _____

MD

From Black, J., and Matassarin-Jacobs, E. [1993]. Luckmann and Sorensen's medical-surgical nursing: A psychophysiologic approach [4th ed.]. Philadelphia: W.B. Saunders.)

CARDIAC MUSCLE CONTRACTION

Match the action potential with the correct phase

33. _____   Phase 0

34. _____   Phase 1

35. _____   Phase 2

36. _____   Phase 3

37. _____   Phase 4

A. Plateau of slow repolarization, potassium leaves cell, sodium enters slowly

B. Sodium is removed, and restoration and initiation of spontaneous diastole occur.

C. Early rapid repolarization occurs as sodium influx stops, potassium leaves cell, chloride enters cell

D. Sodium enters cells rapidly, cells become positive, depolarize and begin to contract.

E. Rapid repolarization occurs as potassium enters and cell becomes negative

CARDIAC CYCLE

Fill in the blanks.

Relaxation period
Occurs at end of (38.)_____
(39.)_____ _____ chambers diastolic
Initiated by repolarization of ventricular muscle fibers
Pressure in chambers drops

Ventricular (45.)_____
Ventricles contract
Semilunar valves (44.)_____ (open/close)
Ventricular pressure increases
Tricuspid and mitral (AV) valves
(43.)_____ (open/close)
Atrial depolarization

Ventricular filling
Tricuspid and mitral (AV) valves
(40.)_____ (open/close)
Semilunar valves (41.)_____ (open/close)
Passive filling of ventricles
(42)_____ contraction during end of diastole

MULTIPLE CHOICE

Select the best answer.

46. Which statement is most accurate about the cardiac cycle?
    A. The duration of the cardiac cycle is 7 cycles per minute.
    B. In the normal cardiac cycle, when the atria contract, the ventricles relax.
    C. The normal cardiac output during a cardiac cycle is 4 to 6 liters of blood.
    D. The cardiac cycle refers to the systolic phase of contraction.

47. Which answer best describes cardiac output?
    A. The less the heart is filled during diastole, the greater the force of the contraction.
    B. The parasympathetic nervous system enhances myocardial contractility.
    C. The primary factor determining afterload is resistance in pulmonic and/or systemic vessels.
    D. Cardiac output is based on action potential and ventricular filling.

48. Which examples of ions and humoral substances' effects on circulatory regulation is correct?
    A. Serotonin acts either as a vasodilator or vasoconstrictor.
    B. Angiotensin and vasopressin are vasodilators.
    C. Sodium and bradykinin are arterial constrictors.
    D. Potassium and hydrogen ions are vasoconstrictors.

CRITICAL THINKING ACTIVITY

How would you figure out the stroke volume if you knew the cardiac output and heart rate?

CHAPTER 30
DRUGS THAT AFFECT VASCULAR TONE

DEFINITION OF TERMS

Define the following:

1. nitrate tolerance

2. typical angina

3. variant angina

ORGANIC NITRATE PROTOTYPE

Complete the following for nitroglycerin.

Pharmacokinetics

4. Transdermal nitroglycerin has an onset of action within _____ to _____ minutes and a duration of action of approximately _____ to _____ hours.

5. The biologic half-life for nitroglycerin ranges from _____ to _____ minutes.

Pharmacodynamics

6. Nitroglycerin reduces _____ and decreases _____. It lowers _____ pressures and peripheral _____.

ERIPHERAL CEREBRAL VASODILATOR PROTOTYPE

Complete the following for papaverine hydrochloride.

Pharmacokinetics

7. Oral tablets and capsules of papaverine are _____ absorbed from the GI tract.

8. Peak levels of papaverine occurs within _____ to _____ hours.

9. Approximately _____% of the drug is bound to plasma protein.

STUDY QUESTIONS

10. Explain the action of organic nitrates that is responsible for relieving angina pectoris.

11. Explain why the oral dosage form of nitroglycerin is not recommended.

12. How many doses of nitroglycerin should an individual take for a single episode of angina pectoris before contacting the primary care provider? Why?

13. What drug-environmental interactions are possible with nitroglycerin?

14. List points to include in a teaching plan for a client being discharged on sublingual nitroglycerin.

15. Explain the role of ß-adrenergic blockers in the treatment of angina pectoris.

16. Explain why calcium channel blockers are used to treat angina. What are the pharmacodynami
properties of this group of drugs?

MULTIPLE CHOICE

Select the best answer.

17. Nitrates relieve angina pectoris by producing peripheral:
  A. vasoconstriction.
  B. suppression of vessel musculature.
  C. vasodilation.
  D. excitation of vessel musculature.

18. Reflex tachycardia is an expected response to which one of the following drugs?
  A. nitroglycerin
  B. propranolol (Inderal)
  C. atenolol (Tenormin)
  D. verapamil (Isoptin)

19. All antianginal drugs alleviate symptoms by
  A. increasing circulating fluid volume.
  B. slowing electrical impulse conduction through the heart.
  C. producing myocardial oxygen supply and demand balance.
  D. lowering the blood pressure.

20. Which one of the following nitrate prepara
tions or dosage forms has the longest dura
tion of action?
  A. sublingual nitroglycerin
  B. sublingual isosorbide dinitrate
  C. translingual spray of nitroglycerin
  D. transdermal patch of nitroglycerin

CRITICAL THINKING ACTIVITY

You are caring for a client who is being started on sublingual nitroglycerin tablets. The client experiences chest pain whenever he/she is under stress. What is probably the precipitating cause of the angina? What instruction should be given to the client?

Chapter 31
CARDIAC GLYCOSIDES

Definition of Terms

Define the following:

1. aglyone

2. cardiac glycosides

3. congestive heart failure

4. digitalis glycosides

5. digitalizing dose

6. maintenance dose

7. pulse deficit

CARDIAC GLYCOSIDES

Complete the following for digoxin (Lanoxin).

Pharmacokinetics

8. GI absorption of digoxin is a _____ process; the degree of absorption depends on the

   _____ _____ .

9. The rate of absorption of an oral dose is _____ when taken after meals.

10. After administration of a digoxin tablet or capsule, onset of action occurs within _____ to _____

    minutes; peak effects occur in _____ to _____ hours.

11. The biologic half-life for digoxin ranges from _____ to _____ days.

Study Questions

12. The body's response to congestive heart failure consists of three primary compensatory mechanisms. Identify each mechanism and describe the changes this mechanism produces in physiologic functioning.

13. The terms *inotropic, chronotropic,* and *dromotropic* are used to describe heart activity. Define each term and tell how this activity is affected by digitalis.

14. Describe the physiologic effects of cardiac glycosides on each of the following body systems.

    renal system

    autonomic nervous system

    endocrine system

15. Provide the rationale for each of the following interventions.
    As part of the health history, collect a nutritional history on the client receiving cardiac glycosides.
    Rationale:

    Before administering a cardiac glycoside, count the pulse for 1 full minute.
    Rationale:

Teach the client not to take cardiac glycoside concurrent with antacids, antidiarrheal drugs, or laxatives.
Rationale:

Unless the client is receiving a potassium-sparing diuretic, teach him/her to eat high potassium foods.
Rationale:

6. In what situation would digoxin immune Fab be administered? What is the desired response to this drug?

7. In what situations is digitoxin the drug of choice over digoxin?

8. List several noncardiac manifestations of digitalis toxicity.

9. List several cardiac manifestations of digitalis toxicity.

Multiple Choice

Select the best answer.

20. The primary therapeutic use of cardiac glycosides is to treat congestive heart failure by their:
    A. positive chronotropic effects.
    B. positive dromotropic action.
    C. positive inotropic action.
    D. negative pressor effect.

21. Which one of the following drugs is used for short-term treatment of severe congestive heart failure?
    A. amrinone (Inocor)
    B. quinidine sulfate (Quinidex)
    C. digitoxin (Crystodigin)
    D. digoxin immune Fab

22. Which one of the following is a physiologic response to cardiac glycoside?
    A. decreased stroke volume
    B. increased vagal influence
    C. increased release of renin
    D. decreased sodium excretion

23. Prior to administering digoxin, the nurse checks the laboratory reports for the client's serum digoxin level. Since the client's level is 1.25 ng/ml, the nurse should:
    A. withhold the drug and contact the primary care provider.
    B. administer a smaller dose than the prescribed dosage.
    C. administer the prescribed dosage and document his/her actions.
    D. withhold the drug and document his/her actions.

CRITICAL THINKING ACTIVITY

You are caring for a client who is being digitalized. What physiologic changes would indicate that the drug is being effective?

Chapter 32
ANTIARRHYTHMIC DRUGS

Definition of Terms

Match the types of arrhythmias listed in Column A with the appropriate definition in Column B.

Column A

1. _____ asystole
2. _____ atrial flutter
3. _____ third-degree block
4. _____ paroxysmal atrial tachycardia
5. _____ sinus tachycardia
6. _____ first-degree block
7. _____ ventricular tachycardia
8. _____ sinus bradycardia

Column B

A. abnormally fast heart rate >100 beats/minutes

B. three or more ventricular complexes; rate >100 beats/minute

C. heart rate < 60 beats/minute

D. absence of impulse initiation in the heart

E. rapid atrial rate of 220-350 beats/minute

F. complete heart block

G. burst of atrial complexes; rate of 160-220 beats/minute

H. prolonged PR intervals; regular rhythm

Match the drugs listed in Column A with the appropriate classification of antiarrhythmic drugs in Column B.

Column A

9. _____ propranolol
10. _____ quinidine
11. _____ verapamil
12. _____ phenytoin
13. _____ propafenone
14. _____ lidocaine
15. _____ esmolol
16. _____ bretylium
17. _____ flecainide
18. _____ moricizine hydrochloride

Column B

A. Class Ia
B. Class Ib
C. Class Ic
D. Class II
E. Class III
F. Class IV
G. Class I

STUDY QUESTIONS

19. Provide the rationale for the following nursing interventions.
    Inject intravenous preparation of quinidine in a diluted state; inject solution slowly.
    Rationale:

    For the client being discharged on flecainide, review signs and symptoms of CHF.
    Rationale:

    Remind the client receiving propranolol to monitor his or her weight weekly and to report any significant weight gain.
    Rationale:

    Instruct client receiving amiodarone hydrochloride to use a sunscreen product with a skin protection factor of greater than SPF 15.
    Rationale:

20. What antiarrhythmic produces such undesired clinical responses as cinchonism and torsades de pointes? Describe each of these undesired responses and identify related nursing interventions.

21. How is the antiarrhythmic drug, lidocaine, administered? Why?

22. In addition to arrhythmias, what other medical conditions are treated with ß-blockers.

23. List common undesired clinical responses associated with ß-adrenergic blockers. What actions by the drugs produce these responses?

24. In addition to arrhythmias, what other medical conditions are treated with calcium-channel blockers.

25. List common undesired clinical responses associated with calcium-channel blockers. What actions by the drugs produce these responses?

MULTIPLE CHOICE

Select the best answer.

26. Which one of the following statements from a client's record would be most helpful in making a nursing judgement about the safe administration of quinidine?
    A. blood pressure—140/78
    B. respirations—20/minute
    C. adequate platelets
    D. apical-radial pulse—106/100

27. A client is receiving quinidine. The nurse assesses the client to determine the effectiveness of the drug therapy. The expected response to the drug is:
    A. suppression of ectopic atrial beats.
    B. decreased blood pressure.
    C. CNS depression.
    D. increased contractility of cardiac muscle.

28. Which one of the following undesired responses can be caused by lidocaine?
    A. renal failure
    B. bleeding
    C. CNS depression
    D. visual disturbances

29. Which would be the drug of choice if the desired action was to prolong the refractory period in conductive fibers?
    A. atropine
    B. mexiletine
    C. tocainide
    D. quinidine

CRITICAL THINKING ACTIVITY

You are preparing to administer procainamide to a client. The following assessment data is available: serum level 6 µ/ml, apical pulse 86; blood pressure 142/96, and widened QRS complex. Based on this data, what action should you take? Provide the rationale for your actions.

CHAPTER 33
ANTIHYPERTENSIVE DRUGS

DEFINITION OF TERMS

Define the following:

1. essential hypertension

2. monotherapy

3. norepinephrine depletor

4. primary hypertension

5. secondary hypertension

CASE STUDY

Ray Jamieson, a 48-year-old African-American male, is admitted to the emergency department with a blood pressure of 294/158. His wife states he has hypertension but has stopped taking his medication recently. The primary care provider orders sodium nitroprusside 50 mg in 500 mL of 5% DW by IV infusion, titrated to decrease diastolic BP to 100 over one hour.

6. What information must you have before initiating the infusion?

Mr. Jamieson's wife states he has no allergies, is 5 feet 6 inches tall and weighs 150 pounds. Mr. Jamieson is alert and reports a headache and nausea. He has been feeling "bad" for several days. Pulse is 96; respirations are 28. The IV is initiated and is infusing at 5 mL/minute.

7. Is the IV infusion rate safe? Explain. How many mcg/minute is Mr. Jamieson receiving?

In discussing drug therapy with Mr. Jamieson, he states he doesn't like to take the drugs for his blood pressure because they have caused him problems with his sex life.

8. How should you respond to this concern?

9. Why is an ACEI drug, which may have less impact on sexuality, not appropriate for this client?

Study Questions

10. How does methyldopa (Aldomet) lower blood pressure?

11. The most common undesired clinical response to central-acting agents is _____.

12. The central-agent, _____ , can be used transdermally for control of hypertension.

13. List instructions the nurse would give a client using the transdermal system.

14. What is a major concern with abrupt cessation of therapy with central- acting agents?

   What actions should the nurse take with regard to this concern?

15. Ganglionic blocking agents are not used for mild or moderate hypertension because:

16. The dose of mecamylamine (Inversine) is regulated by _____ _____.

17. What interventions can help minimize this effect of alpha$_1$-adrenergic blockers?

18. Identify the generic and brand names for three alpha$_1$-adrenergic blockers.

19. What two population groups respond less well to beta-blockers?

20. List three health problems which, if identified in the nursing history, would be relative or absolut contraindications for treatment with beta blockers.

21. Labetalol hydrochloride (Normodyne, Trandate) can be administered intravenously in hypertensiv urgencies or emergencies. Explain nursing actions related to the IV infusion.

22. Rauwolfia alkaloids are classified as _____.

23. Why is use of rauwolfia alkaloids limited?

24. Identify quality of life side effects that limit use of norepinephrine depletors in general.

25. Why is monitoring of pulse of particular importance with administration of direct vasodilators

26. Hydralazine hydrochloride (Apresoline) is used to treat _____
     and _____.

27. What is the recommended IV infusion rate of diazoxide (Hyperstat)?

28. What is the "minibolus" dose of diazoxide?

29. What is the primary difference in first and second generation calcium-channel blockers?

0. Explain the action of ACEI agents.

1. List the most common undesired effects of ACEI drugs.

Match the drug on the left to the commonly associated undesired response on the right.

2. ____   reserpine

3. ____   methyldopa

4. ____   enalapril

5. ____   mecamylamine

6. ____   prazosin

7. ____   hydralazine

A. syncope, first-dose effect

B. adynamic ileus

C. sedation

D. reflexive tachycardia

E. cough

F. depression

MULTIPLE CHOICE

Select the best answer.

8. Diazoxide (Hyperstat) is administered by IV infusion. The nurse would consider adequate blood pressure reduction to be reached when the diastolic pressure is less than:
    A. 150 mg
    B. 100 mg
    C. 90 mg
    D. 80 mg

9. The nurse monitors a diazoxide infusion carefully because extravasation causes:
    A. cellulitis.
    B. flare reaction.
    C. thrombophlebitis.
    D. allergic wheals.

40. Angiotensin-converting enzyme inhibitors (ACEI) are least effective in which of the following population groups:
    A. Orientals
    B. Caucasians
    C. African-Americans
    D. women

41. The nurse advises the client who is receiving lisinopril (Prinivil, Zestril) of its most common undesired clinical responses, including:
    A. sedation and dry mouth.
    B. sodium and water retention.
    C. palpitations and flushing.
    D. headache, nausea, and vomiting.

CRITICAL THINKING ACTIVITY

If an individual has hypertension, what is the danger of taking an OTC drug containing phenylephrine (a mixed acting adrenergic drug)?

CHAPTER 34
DRUGS AFFECTING PLASMA LIPIDS AND COAGULATION FACTORS

DEFINITION OF TERMS

Define the following:

1. agglutination

2. aggregation

3. antithrombin III

4. extrinsic pathway

5. intrinsic pathway

6. plasmin

7. plasminogen

8. plasminogen activators

9. platelet degranulation

10. white-clot syndrome

STUDY QUESTIONS

11. Describe the hemostatic process. Consider the following aspects: mechanisms of hemostasis; th coagulation process; role of vitamin K in coagulation; and countermechanisms to blood clotting

12. Describe each of the following diagnostic tests and indicate their relationship to drug therapy

    prothrombin time

    partial thromboplastin time

    aspirin-tolerance test

    bleeding time test

    total cholesterol levels

    lipoprotein fractionation

13. Develop a teaching plan for clients receiving antilipidemic drug therapy. Consider pharmacoki netic and pharmacodynamic properties and undesired clinical responses of the drugs whe preparing the plan.

14. Describe the anticoagulant actions of heparin.

15. What diagnostic test is used when determining heparin dosages?

6. Describe the SC injection technique to be used when administering heparin. What is the preferred site for this injection?

7. Describe the physiologic action of warfarin sodium.

8. What diagnostic test is used to determine warfarin dosage?

9. What drugs interact with heparin? with warfarin?

10. What is the antidote for heparin? for warfarin?

11. Develop a teaching plan for a client receiving oral anticoagulant drug therapy. Consider drug-drug, drug-nutrient, and drug-environment interactions when preparing the plan.

12. Mark each of the following statements with an H for heparin and a W for warfarin. If the statement is correct for both drugs, use HW.

_____ Half life approximately 1 to 2 hours

_____ Onset of action in 12 to 72 hours

_____ Can cause hemorrhaging

_____ Effects persist for 24 to 96 hours

_____ Laxatives decrease absorption rate

_____ Can interact with aspirin

ANTILIPIDEMIC DRUGS

Complete the following:

23. Bile acid sequestrant resins act by _____

_____.

They also promote _____catabolism. Common undesired responses to these drugs include:

_____.

24. Nicotinic acid is a _____-soluble vitamin. Its exact mechanism of action is not known.

_____ _____ is a prominent undesired response associated

with nicotinic acid.

25. HMG-CoA reductase inhibitors act by _____

Drugs included in this group include: _____

_____.

ANTIPLATELET DRUGS

Complete the following:

26. Aspirin is the prototype antiplatelet drug. It prevents the _____

which is necessary for maximum _____ _____.

THROMBOLYTIC DRUGS

Complete the following:

27. The prototype first-generation thrombolytic drug is _____. This

drug acts by _____. The

most dangerous adverse effect to this drug is _____

MULTIPLE CHOICE

Select the best answer

28. The conversion of protein prothrombin to thrombin occurs during which phase of blood clotting?
    A. Phase I
    B. Phase II
    C. Phase III
    D. Phase IV

29. The anticoagulant action of heparin includes:
    A. interfering with the action of vitamin K.
    B. forming an inactive complex with calcium.
    C. destruction of thrombin and activated Factor X.
    D. lysis of existing thrombus.

30. Heparin can be administered by each of the following methods *except*:
    A. intramuscular
    B. intravenous infusion
    C. subcutaneous
    D. intravenous bolus

31. Cholestyramine (Questran) comes in a powder form. It:
    A. can be safely administered within 30 minutes of other medications.
    B. can be safely administered at the same time as other drugs.
    C. is sprinkled on the surface of dry food.
    D. is sprinkled on the surface of liquid or semiliquid food.

CRITICAL THINKING ACTIVITY

You are preparing to administer a dose of heparin. You note that the client's clotting time is 12 minutes and his partial thromboplastin time is 53 seconds. His last heparin was administered 5 hours ago. What actions should you take?

CHAPTER 35

OVERVIEW OF THE RENAL SYSTEM

DEFINITION OF TERMS

Define the following:

1. angiotensin II

2. diffusion

3. filtrate

4. filtration

5. hydrostatic pressure

6. osmosis

7. osmotic pressure

8. tubular reabsorption

9. tubular secretion

From the list of transport mechanisms in Column B, select one or more mechanisms for the exchange of substances (Column A) between the tubular filtrate and the blood:

Column A		Column B	
10. _____	sodium ions	A.	active transport
11. _____	chloride	B.	filtration
12. _____	potassium ions	C.	passive transport
13. _____	glucose	D.	reabsorption
14. _____	secretion	E.	secretion

STUDY QUESTIONS

15. What is the function of ADH (antidiuretic hormone)?

16. Briefly describe the composition of urine.

17. What is the function of aldosterone?

18. What are the major functions of the renal system?

19. Describe the role of the renal system in regulation of hydrogen ion balance.

20. Describe the role of the renal system in regulation of calcium and phosphate balance.

21. Describe the regulation of GFR. Consider renal autoregulation, neural regulation, and hormonal regulation.

MULTIPLE CHOICE

Select the best answer.

22. The functional units of the kidney are the:
    A. collecting tubules.
    B. calyces.
    C. nephrons.
    D. capillaries.

23. The urine collecting portion of the kidney is the renal:
    A. cortex.
    B. medulla.
    C. capsule.
    D. pelvis.

24. The kidney and urinary bladder are connected by the:
    A. collecting tubules.
    B. calyx.
    C. urethra.
    D. ureter.

Chapter 36
DIURETICS

Definition of Terms

Define the following:

1. aldosterone antagonist

2. aquaretics

3. diuretic

4. hypochloremic alkalosis

5. kaliuretic

6. natriuretic

7. nonaldosterone antagonist

8. solute diuretic

9. water diuretic

Match the undesired clinical responses in Column A with the appropriate condition in Column B. Response may have more than one answer.

	Column A		Column B
10. _____	tetany	A.	hyponatremia
11. _____	tingling of ends of fingers	B.	hypovolemia
12. _____	intestinal colic	C.	hypokalemia
13. _____	decreased intestinal function	D.	hyperkalemia
14. _____	deep bone pain	E.	metabolic alkalosis
15. _____	hyperactive deep tendon reflexes	F.	hypocalcemia
16. _____	confusion	G.	hypercalcemia
17. _____	body weight loss	H.	hypomagnesemia
18. _____	convulsions		
19. _____	diarrhea		
20. _____	longitudinal tongue wrinkles		

THIAZIDE DIURETICS

Complete the following for hydrochlorothiazide (Hydrodiuril, Esidrix).

Pharmacokinetics

21. Hydrochlorothiazide is _____ absorbed from the GI tract and produces diuretic

    effects within _____ hours.

    Peak effect usually occurs in approximately _____ hours and lasts approximately _____ to _____

    hours.

    The plasma half-life for hydrochlorothiazide is _____ to _____ hours.

    At least _____% of an oral dose is eliminated unchanged within 24 hours.

Pharmacodynamics

22. Hydrochlorothiazide acts on the _____ _____ _____

    to inhibit _____ and _____ reabsorption. Therapeutic doses of

    thiazides increase urinary _____ and _____excretion.

23. Hydrochlorothiazide significantly _____ renal tubular secretion of _____

    _____, increasing the client's potential for gout.

LOOP DIURETICS

Complete the following for furosemide (Lasix).

Pharmacokinetics

24. Furosemide is _____absorbed from the GI tract. Its protein binding is greater than _____%

    Onset of action with oral dosage occurs within _____ to _____ minutes; peak action occurs in _____

    to _____ hours; duration of action is _____ to _____hours.

25. Onset of action following IV injection is approximately _____ minutes; duration of action is _____

    to _____ hours.

OSMOTIC DIURETICS

Complete the following for mannitol (Osmitrol, Mannitol).

Pharmacokinetics

26. Mannitol is _____ distributed to extracellular fluid after IV administration

    Diuresis occurs in _____ to _____ hours; peak effect in _____to _____ minutes; duration of action

    is _____ to _____ hours.

Pharmacodynamics

7. Mannitol is a _____ solute that acts along the entire nephron. It induces diuresis by elevating the _____ of the glomerular filtrate, hindering tubular reabsorption of _____ and increasing excretion of _____ and _____.

STUDY QUESTIONS

8. Identify which classification of diuretics acts on each of the following sites:
   a.   Proximal convoluted tubule:

   b.   Ascending limb of the loop of Henle:

   c.   Distal convoluted tubule:

   d.   Terminal distal convoluted tubule:

   e.   Cortical collecting duct:

9. Explain the term *contraction alkalosis*

30. Mrs. S., a 54-year-old African-American, has been followed for several years for chronic renal problems. She is currently being seen for reevaluation of her drug regime. She leaves the clinic with prescriptions for Corgard 40 mg daily, Lasix 40 mg bid, and Di-Gel 5 ml as needed.

    Supply the generic name for each of these drugs.

    Explain the pharmacotherapeutic, pharmacokinetic, and pharmacodynamic properties of each drug.

    Identify and describe any potential drug-drug or drug-food interactions.

    List one appropriate nursing diagnosis and related nursing interventions.

31. Provide rationale for the following interventions.
    Teach client to take once-daily doses of diuretics early in the day, shortly after awakening.
    Rationale:

    Discuss with the client the importance of reducing dietary intake of sodium.
    Rationale:

Teach the client the major signs and symptoms of hypokalemia.
Rationale:

Tell client to weigh daily, preferably upon arising, after voiding, and before eating.
Rationale:

Carefully monitor the client's fluid intake and urinary output.
Rationale:

MULTIPLE CHOICE

Select the best answer.

32. Diuretics can be used to treat hypertension. At maximally effective doses, diuretics:
    A. enhance tubular sodium reabsorption.
    B. reduce blood pressure about 15 mm Hg.
    C. lower blood pressure in normotensive individuals.
    D. enhance tubular reabsorption of potassium.

33. You should assess all clients receiving thiazide diuretics for hypokalemia. Which one of the following might indicate hypokalemia:
    A. headaches
    B. muscle weakness
    C. dehydration
    D. hypertension

34. When a thiazide diuretic is administered, you should encourage the client to drink additional amounts of:
    A. milk.
    B. coffee.
    C. fruit juice.
    D. tea.

35. Your assessment of a client reveals: apical, radical pulse—58/58; serum potassium —3.3 mEq/l; blood pressure—86/46. Based on this information, which one of the following drugs could you safely administer without notifying the primary care provider or obtaining additional information?
    A. digoxin
    B. hydrochlorothiazide
    C. potassium chloride
    D. furosemide (Lasix)

36. The client is to be discharged with a prescription for triamterene, a potassium-sparing diuretic. The nurse should teach the client to:
    A. include foods high in potassium in his/her diet.
    B. include foods high in sodium in his/her diet.
    C. avoid foods high in potassium.
    D. avoid foods high in magnesium.

CRITICAL THINKING ACTIVITY

What affects do thiazide diuretics have on uric acid and calcium?

What potential medical problem might this produce and what could you, the nurse, do to prevent this problem?

Chapter 37
HYPERURICEMIC DRUGS

Definition of Terms

Define the following:

1. acute gout

2. asymptomatic hyperuricemia

3. gout

4. hyperuricemia

5. purine

6. tophaceous gout

7. tophi

8. urate

URICOSURIC PROTOTYPE

Complete the following for probenecid (Benemid).

Pharmacokinetics

9. Probenecid is _____ absorbed from the GI tract.

   Peak plasma levels are reached in _____ to _____ hours.

   The plasma half-life for probenecid is _____ to _____ hours.

Pharmacodynamics

10. Probenecid inhibits tubular reabsorption of _____, thus increasing the urinary

    excretion of _____ _____. Therapeutic doses of probenecid can

    _____ urate excretion in clients with gout.

URIC ACID SYNTHESIS INHIBITOR DIURETICS

Complete the following for allopurinol (Zyloprim).

Pharmacokinetics

11. Allopurinol is _____ absorbed from the GI tract. Its half-life is _____ to _____

hours. Its active metabolite, _____ has a half-life of _____ to _____ hours.

Undesired Clinical Responses

12. Undesired clinical responses to allopurinol are more severe than those responses associated with

other uricosuric drugs. The most common response is _____. Other common

responses include: _____.

STUDY QUESTIONS

13. Describe the process of uric acid synthesis.

14. Describe the process of renal excretion of uric acid.

15. Provide rationale for the following interventions.
Teach client the importance of avoiding alcohol and salicylates when receiving hyperuricemic drugs.
Rationale:

Advise the client to ingest at least 2 to 3 L of fluid per day.
Rationale:

Teach the client to avoid drinking vitamin C preparations or juices such as cranberry juice.
Rationale:

Carefully monitor the client's fluid intake and urinary output.
Rationale:

When appropriate, teach client to avoid high-purine foods and caffeine.
Rationale:

16. Which of the following—probenecid, allopurinol, or colchicine—is used to treat acute gouty arthritis? Why is it the drug of choice in this situation?

MULTIPLE CHOICE

Select the best answer.

17. A client is to begin colchicine. The nurse will anticipate the following dosage schedule:
    A. hourly until pain is reduced
    B. hourly during the acute phase
    C. every 2 hours during the acute phase
    D. every 4 hours during the maintenance phase

18. The client is receiving allopurinol 300 mg orally daily. It is important for the client to:
    A. avoid exposure to sunlight.
    B. avoid strenuous exercise.
    C. increase fluid intake.
    D. increase intake of protein foods.

19. Uricosuric drugs such as probenecid act by:
    A. decreasing the activity of leukocytes.
    B. stimulating the breakdown of purine in the liver.
    C. inhibiting the conversion of xanthine to uric acid.
    D. inhibiting the tubular reabsorption of uric acid.

20. When evaluating the client's response to therapy with allopurinol, the best clinical indicator would be:
    A. serum uric acid levels.
    B. serum calcium and phosphorous levels.
    C. urinary urate content.
    D. white blood cell count and differential.

CRITICAL THINKING ACTIVITY

A client comes to the clinic with complaints of pain in the right great toe. The affected joint is hot, red, and extremely tender. What is the drug of choice to treat the client's current condition? Why?

A client is receiving a thiazide diuretic for treatment of hypertension. His/her serum uric acid level becomes elevated. What is the drug of choice to treat the client's condition? Why?

CHAPTER 38
OVERVIEW OF THE ENDOCRINE SYSTEM

DEFINITION OF TERMS

HORMONES

Match the description with the term.

1. _____ Circulating hormones

2. _____ Local hormones

3. _____ Steroid hormones

4. _____ Biogenic amines

5. _____ Peptides and proteins

6. _____ Eicosanoids

A. Hormones that act on target cells close to the site of release.

B. The most recently discovered hormones. Example: prostaglandins.

C. The simplest hormone molecules. Example: Thyroxine.

D. Hormones that pass into the blood and act on distant target cells.

E. Hormones consisting of chains of amino acids. Example: insulin.

F. Hormones derived from cholesterol. Example: cortisol.

HYPOTHALAMUS AND PITUITARY GLAND

PITUITARY

For each pituitary hormone, match the principal action.

7. _____   Thyroid-stimulating hormone (TSH)

8. _____   Adrenocorticotropic hormone (ACTH)

9. _____   Melanocyte-stimulating hormone (MSH)

10. _____   Growth hormone (GH)

11. _____   Follicle-stimulating hormone (FSH)

12. _____   Leutenizing hormone (LH)

13. _____   Prolactin

14. _____   Oxytocin

15. _____   Antidiuretic hormone

A.   Stimulates contraction of uterus during labor and mammary glands for milk ejection

B.   Growth of body cells

C.   Initiates development of ova and secretion of estrogens in females; stimulates sperm production in males

D.   Stimulates dispersion of melanin granules in melanocytes

E.   Decreases urinary volume, raises blood pressure

F.   Promotes milk secretion by mammary glands

G.   Controls secretion of adrenal cortical hormones

H.   Controls secretion of thyroid hormones

I.   Stimulates ovulation in females and testosterone production in males

THYROID GLAND AND PARATHYROID GLAND

Indicate if the statement is true or false. Correct the false statements.

16. _____   Release of thyroid hormones is regulated primarily by positive feedback.

17. _____   When circulating levels of T_3 and T_4 become too low, the hypothalamus releases TRH which stimulates the anterior pituitary lobe to secrete TSH.

18. _____   Thyroid hormones decrease the basal metabolic rate (BMR), thus decreasing the rate of protein, carbohydrate, lipid, and vitamin metabolism.

19. _____   Thyroid hormones decrease the permeability of cell membranes to sodium and potassium.

20. _____   Parafollicular cells produce calcitonin only when there is decreased calcium in the blood

21. _____ Parathormone increases calcium and phosphate absorption from the bone and decreases renal excretion of calcium.

22. _____ Parathormone promotes the formation of the hormone calcitonin.

23. _____ Calcitriol increases serum calcium and magnesium concentrations and maintain normal phosphate levels.

PANCREAS

Complete by circling the correct words.

Glucagon	Insulin
Secreted by (24.) *alpha/beta* cells	Secreted by (25.) *alpha/beta* cells
Peptide hormone	Peptide hormone
(26.) *Raises/Lowers* blood glucose level	(27.) *Raises/Lowers* blood glucose level
	Makes cell membranes (28.) *less/more* permeable to amino acids and electrolytes such as potassium, magnesium, and phosphates
	Essential for protein (29.)*catabolism/synthesis* and (30.) *mobilization/storage*
	Stimulates adipose cells to (31.)*catabolize/ synthesize* and (32.) *mobilize/ store* fat.
Action: (33.) *accelerates/decreases* conversion of glycogen to glucose Also promotes conversion of other nutrients into glucose in liver (34.) *gluconeogenesis/glycogenesis*.	Action: acts on liver to (35.) *inhibit/stimulate* formation of glycogen from glucose and to inhibit conversion of non-carbohydrates into glucose.
	Also accelerates (36.) *transport/storage* of glucose into cells that possess insulin receptors.
	Promotes (37.) *transport/storage* of amino acids into cells and (38.) *increases/decreases* synthesis of proteins.
	Required for conversion of glucose to triglycerides, which are stored as adipose tissue

CRITICAL THINKING ACTIVITY

Which category of corticosteroids is essential to life? Why?

CHAPTER 39
DRUGS USED TO REGULATE BLOOD GLUCOSE LEVELS

DEFINITION OF TERMS

Define the following:

1. dawn phenomenon

2. flocculation

3. glucagon

4. hyperglycemia

5. hyperinsulinism

6. hypoglycemia

7. insulin resistance

8. ketoacidosis

9. ketone bodies

10. lipohypertrophy

11. lipotrophy

12. postprandial hypoglycemia

13. renal threshold

14. somatostatin

MANAGEMENT OF DIABETES MELLITUS

Determine if each diabetic teaching statement is true or false. Correct the false statements.

5. _____ If you start to feel shaky, sweaty, or lightheaded, you are having a hypoglycemic reaction. You need to take some carbohydrates in order to prevent damage to your pancreas.

6. _____ Since you have insulin-dependent diabetes mellitus, your pancreas continues to make insulin, but the insulin is ineffective. You will need to take an oral hypoglycemic drug daily to correct this problem.

7. _____ Since insulin is a hormone, it must always be stored in a refrigerator to prevent loss of potency.

8. _____ When you exercise, do it shortly before the next meal and decrease your insulin dosage by 15 units.

9. _____ Be sure to rotate the site of your insulin injections. This is done to avoid damage to the tissues.

10. _____ Since you are mixing regular and NPH insulins together, it is important to always draw up the regular insulin first.

11. _____ Testing your urine for glucose is the most accurate measurement for diabetic control.

12. _____ Do not use insulin that has sediment in the bottom of the vial or appears cloudy.

13. _____ It is all right to change brands of insulin, but do not ever change preparations or potency without consulting your primary care provider.

INSULIN

Match the type of insulin with the characteristics. You will have 5 answers for each type of insulin and you may use the answers more than one time.

24. ____   Short acting

25. ____   Intermediate acting

26. ____   Long acting

A.   Most rapid onset, within 30 to 60 minutes

B.   Seldom used alone

C.   Regular insulin combined with protamine or zinc

D.   Administered only subcutaneously

E.   Shortest duration of action, 3 to 6 hours

F.   Hypoglycemia most likely in late afternoon

G.   Eating a bedtime snack will help prevent decreased blood glucose while sleeping

H.   Duration of action generally longer than 24 hours

I.   May be given by the intravenous route

J.   Includes NPH and Lente insulin

K.   Includes Ultralente and protamine zinc

L.   Includes regular and semilente insulin

M.   Used for diabetic emergencies

Match the drug with the description. There are two answers for each drug.

27. ____   Glyburide

28. ____   Glipizide

29. ____   Acetohexamide

30. ____   Chlorpropamide

31. ____   Tolazamide

32. ____   Tolbutamide

A.   Useful to clients with congestive heart failure, hepatic cirrhosis, and fluid retention.

B.   Few serious side effects. Common side effect is nausea.

C.   The drug to avoid if the client is elderly.

D.   The drug that is safe with elderly clients

E.   Presence of foods delay absorption.

F.   The only one with uricosuric properties.

G.   First generation

H.   Second generation

RUGS TO INCREASE BLOOD GLUCOSE LEVELS

Complete the sentences by unscrambling the words.

3. Glucagon can be used to treat insulin (Tenacosir)_____or

   (Mopecygilyha) _____ in diabetic clients.

4. Synthetic glucagon must be administered (Lerytenalarp)_____.

5. Undesired clinical responses to glucagon are (Shar) _____ , dizziness, nausea, vomiting,

   and (Polemykahia) _____.

6. Diabetics are encouraged to carry this drug with them at all times. (Sucogel) _____.

7. (Xazidoid) _____ inhibits insulin secretion.

8. The prototype hypoglycemia antagonist is (Nogaculg) _____.

MULTIPLE CHOICE

Select the best answer.

9. Insulin-dependent diabetes mellitus (IDDM) differs from non-insulin-dependent diabetes mellitus (NIDDM) in what way?
   A. IDDM is caused by ineffective function of insulin; NIDDM is caused insufficient insulin production.
   B. IDDM usually occurs gradually, NIDDM usually occurs abruptly.
   C. IDDM is the most frequently occurring type of diabetes; NIDDM only occurs in about 10% of the population.
   D. Clinical manifestations of IDDM are more severe than NIDDM.

0. Which answer best describes correct insulin administration?
   A. Absorption is most complete when administered in the upper body (arms).
   B. It is recommended to move to a different anatomic location (example, arm, leg) for each injection.
   C. The most common method of insulin delivery is intramuscular injection at a 45 degree angle.
   D. It is recommended to allow $1/2$ to 1 inch between injection sites in an anatomic location.

41. Which factor would decrease sc insulin absorption?
    A. exercise
    B. injection in abdomen
    C. smoking
    D. eating a high carbohydrate meal

42. Which sentence about types of insulins is correct?
    A. Administer short acting insulin at least two hours before a meal.
    B. NPH and Lente insulins should be used for diabetic emergencies.
    C. Lente insulins should only be mixed with Lente preparations.
    D. Human regular insulin and ultralente insulin should never be mixed.

CRITICAL THINKING ACTIVITY

If a client is going for a 10 mile run, where should the insulin be injected? Why?

CHAPTER 40

DRUGS AFFECTING HYPOTHALAMIC AND PITUITARY FUNCTIONS

DEFINITION OF TERMS

Define the following:

1. adrenocorticotropin

2. diabetes insipidus

3. primary adrenocortical deficiency

4. secondary adrenocortical deficiency

STUDY QUESTIONS

5. Explain two reasons why there are limited or no approved clinical uses for hypothalamic and pituitary hormones.

6. List three therapeutic uses for corticotropin.

7. You are caring for a client on long-term corticotropin therapy. For each of the following bod systems, describe the related undesired clinical responses and appropriate nursing measure

Central nervous system:

Cardiovascular system:

Urinary system:

Endocrine system:

Integumentary system:

PROTOTYPE DRUGS AFFECTING THE ENDOCRINE SYSTEM

Fill in the blank with the appropriate drug—Corticotropin, Somatrem, or Vasopressin

	Pharmacotherapeutics	
8. _____	9. _____	10. _____
Treatment of diabetes insipidus caused by nonproduction of natural ADH Relief of postoperative intestinal gas distention Adjunct treatment of acute, massive hemorrhage caused by ruptured areas in the GI tract	Diagnosis of adrenocorticoid function Treat conditions responsive to glucocorticoid therapy: exacerbations of multiple sclerosis, rheumatic disorders, collagen diseases, allergic reactions, leukemias, lymphomas, and ulcerative colitis	Used to increase growth rate in clients with growth failure or delayed physiologic development due to insufficient endogenous growth hormone secretion Not effective for impaired growth from other causes or after puberty

Pharmacokinetics

11. _____	12. _____	13. _____
Serum levels highest with SC abdominal injection.	Destroyed by trypsin in GI tract	Destroyed by proteolytic enzymes in digestive tract
Individual absorption rates vary.	Distributed throughout extracellular fluid after parenteral administration	Rapidly removed from plasma by many tissues after injection
Bound to high-affinity growth hormone-binding protein	Onset of action 1 minute after IV administration	Onset action of 5 minutes
Half-life is 2–3 hours	Duration 2–8 hours after SC and 6–12 after IV administration	Duration of 2–4 hours
Metabolized in liver and excreted in kidneys, more rapidly in adults		Half-life < 20 minutes

Contraindications and Precautions

14. _____	15. _____	16. _____
Hypersensitivity to the drug	Cushing's syndrome	Precarious fluid and electrolyte balance
Clients with closed epiphyses or actively growing intracranial lesions	Diabetes mellitus	Preoperative and postoperative polyuria clients
Family history of diabetes	Psychotic or psychopathic disorders	Renal disease
Hypothyroid clients	Active tuberculosis	Comatose clients
Pregnancy Category C drug	Acquired immune deficiency syndrome	Pregnant women
	Live vaccine immunization	Bowel obstruction
	Allergies to pork products	Heart disease
	Hypertension and congestive heart failure	
	Myasthenia gravis	
	Preganancy Category C drug	

CRITICAL THINKING ACTIVITY

Walter B., age 9, has been diagnosed with growth failure due to lack of endogenous growth hormone. His physician prescribed Somatrem (Protropin) 0.1 mg/kg body weight three times per week.

What assessment is essential before therapy is initiated?

What teaching should occur with Walter? His family?

How many milligrams of Somatrem will the client receive each dose?

Mr. James Walker, age 24, has been involved in an automobile accident, resulting in serious head injury. Over the last eight hours Mr. Walker has had more than 2400cc of urine output. His skin is dry, he has poor skin turgor, and his mucous membranes are dry. Upon reporting these findings, vasopressin 10 U IM bid is ordered.

What medical condition do these signs and symptoms suggest?

What baseline values are important before initiating drug therapy with vasopressin?

What physiologic changes should occur following administration of the drug?

The nurse should monitor for what undesired clinical responses during therapy?

CHAPTER 41
DRUGS AFFECTING THYROID AND PARATHYROID FUNCTIONS

DEFINITION OF TERMS

Define the following:

1. calcitonin

2. hyperparathyroidism

3. hypoparathyroidism

4. hyperthyroidism

5. hypothyroidism

6. parathormone

7. thyroiditis

8. thyroxine

9. triiodothyronine

HYROID HORMONE REPLACEMENT PROTOTYPE

Complete the following for levothyroxine sodium (Eltroxin, Levothroid, Synthroid).

Pharmacokinetics

0. After oral administration, levothyroxine has variable absorption, _____ to _____ %, from the GI tract.

1. Highest concentration of the drug occurs in the _____ and _____.

2. Levothyroxine has a slow onset and long duration of action. The plasma half-life is _____ to _____ days; full effects of drug may not occur for _____ to _____ weeks.

Pharmacodynamics

13. Levothyroxine sodium binds to receptors throughout the body,_____ th

    metabolic rate of body tissues. It promotes _____, stimulate

    protein synthesis, and promotes cell _____ and _____

ANTITHYROID DRUG PROTOTYPE

Complete the following for propylthiouracil.

Pharmacokinetics

14. After oral administration, propylthiouracil is _____ absorbed.

15. Therapeutic effects begin within ____ minutes. The plasma half-life is ____ hours.

Pharmacodynamics

16. Propylthiouracil _____; i
    does not inhibit action of thyroid hormones already formed.

CALCIUM REGULATOR PROTOTYPE

Complete the following for calcitonin.

Pharmacokinetics

17. Calcitonin must be administered _____.

18. Onset of action after IM or SC administration is ____ minutes. Peak action occurs in ____ hours

    and duration of action is ____ hours.

Pharmacodynamics

19. When calcitonin is administered, the serum level of _____ is lowered and urinar

    excretion of _____, _____, and _____ increases

STUDY QUESTIONS

20. For each of the body systems listed, provide three undesired responses to drugs used to trea
    thyroid deficiency.

    a.   central nervous system

    b.   endocrine system

    c.   integumentary system

    d.   cardiovascular system

    e.   autonomic nervous system

1. Provide rationales for the following interventions.
   Administer levothyroxine sodium at the same time each day.
   Rationale:

   Monitor the client's pulse for rate and rhythm during initial therapy with levothyroxine.
   Rationale:

   Levothyroxine must be used with extreme caution in clients with angina.
   Rationale:

2. What information is critical to the teaching plan of a client receiving levothyroxine sodium?

3. Explain precautions associated with administration of levothyroxine to pregnant women and their infants.

4. Identify five drugs that interact with levothyroxine.

5. Identify therapeutic uses for radioactive iodine.

6. Describe precautions used with clients receiving radioactive iodine for either hyperthyroidism or cancer of the thyroid.

CRITICAL THINKING ACTIVITY

Julie Oberknecht, age 20, has been suffering from symptoms of hypothyroidism including excessive sedation, bradycardia, hypotension, and intolerance of cold. T_3, T_4, and TSH levels are ordered.

What laboratory values would be consistent with the client's clinical manifestations?

Levothyroxine sodium, 50 micrograms daily for one week, is prescribed and then the laboratory tests repeated. What changes should be reflected in the repeat diagnostic studies?

During the second week of therapy, the dosage is increased to 75 micrograms daily. What indicates that a therapeutic dosage has been reached?

CHAPTER 42

ADRENAL CORTICOIDS

DEFINITION OF TERMS

Match the term with the correct definition.

1. _____ Adrenocortical hormones

2. _____ Androgens

3. _____ Glucocorticoids

4. _____ Mineralocorticoids

5. _____ Cushingoid appearance

6. _____ Adrenal insufficiency

7. _____ Adrenal suppression

A. An adrenocortical hormone that maintains fluid and electrolyte balance.

B. Impaired corticoid production by the adrenal gland.

C. Hormones synthesized and secreted by the adrenal cortex.

D. An adrenocortical hormone that possesses antiinflammatory and immunosuppressive properties.

E. Decreased stimulation for adrenal functioning.

F. An adrenocortical hormone that produces masculinizing effects.

G. A pattern of fat deposits from glucocorticoids resulting in a buffalo hump and moon face.

GLUCOCORTICOID DRUGS

PHARMACOTHERAPEUTICS

Fill in the blanks for the primary uses of glucocorticoid drugs.

8. Replacement therapy for primary_____ _____
   (Addison's disease) or _____ _____ insufficiency.

9. _____ therapy.

10. Anti _____ therapy.

11. _____ distress syndrome in preterm infants.

Complete the blanks with the common undesired clinical responses associated with glucocorticoid drugs.

Central Nervous System

12. Steroid induced _____

Sensory System
Cataract development

13. _____

Gastrointestinal System

14. _____ _____ formation

Endocrine System

15. _____ appetite

16. _____ caloric intake

17. Mobilization of _____

18. _____ deposits of fats

19. _____ glycemia

20. _____ tissue use of glucose

21. _____ of muscle protein

22. Adrenal _____

23. _____ insufficiency

Urinary System

24. _____ retention

25. _____ excretion

26. Water _____

Musculoskeletal System

27. Interference with _____ balance

28. _____

29. Muscle _____

30. Loss of _____ mass

evelop a nursing care plan using three of the nursing diagnoses for clients on long-term
lucocorticoid therapy (see p. 528 of the text).

Nursing Diagnosis and Expected Outcomes	Interventions
Nursing diagnosis #1 Goal: Expected Outcomes:	
Nursing diagnosis #2 Goal: Expected Outcomes:	
Nursing diagnosis #3 Goal: Expected Outcomes:	

PREDNISONE—GLUCOCORTICOID PROTOTYPE

FLUDROCORTISONE ACETATE—MINERALOCORTICOID PROTOTYPE

Complete the following table by filling in the missing words. The first letter is provided for you

Prednisone	Fludrocortisone Acetate
Pharmacotherapeutics	
31. A_____ deficiency states; COPD; r_____ a_____; allergic rhinitis; asthma; pneumocystis pneumonia; ulcerative colitis, Crohn's disease; and cluster headaches	32. Primary and secondary a_____ insufficiency in Addison's disease (combined with glucocorticoids); and salt-losing adrenogenital syndrome
Pharmacokinetics	
33. Readily absorbed from G___ _____	Readily absorbed from GI tract
34. Metabolized in liver where converted to active form, p_____ Excreted by kidneys.	35. Excreted by k_____
Pharmacodynamics	
36. Prednisolone (active form) binds to g_____ receptor sites. 37. Bound receptor sites change form and bind to DNA and cell nucleus p_____ . Changes in levels of proteins cause physiologic effects on clients. 38. I_____ response altered by decreasing T-helper lymphocyte populations, antibody synthesis, and formation of immune complexes. 39. Inflammatory response altered because of interference of essential events of I_____ process.	40. Combines with receptor sites in target cells competing with g_____ . 41. Act on r_____ distal tubules to enhance reabsorption of sodium and c_____ ions and excretion of p_____ and and hydrogen ions.
Pharmaceutics	
Tablets, oral solution, oral syrup	Tablets

MULTIPLE CHOICE

Select the best answer.

2. Besides their antiinflammatory and immunosuppressant properties, other properties
of glucocorticoids are:
   A. They influence carbohydrate, lipid, and
   protein metabolism.
   B. They are produced in decreased
   amounts during stressful times and
   exercise.
   C. They increase serum calcium levels
   by redistributing intracellular calcium.
   D. They stimulate defense mechanisms
   to produce inflammation and immunity.

3. Which statement is most accurate about
administering glucocorticoid therapy? Glucocorticoids:
   A. are usually administered in the early
   evening to coincide with the natural
   secretion pattern of the adrenal
   glands.
   B. are usually administered on a strict,
   unchanging schedule.
   C. may be administered with food to decrease gastric irritation.
   D. are not administered intravenously
   because of serious risks associated with
   this form of delivery.

44. Which answer is correct about glucocorticoid drugs?
   A. Hydrocortisone and cortisone are examples of long acting drugs.
   B. Prednisolone is intermediate acting and
   given to clients unable to metabolize
   prednisone.
   C. Dexamethasone and betamethasone are
   examples of short acting drugs.
   D. Prednisone and prednisolone are inter-
   changeable drugs.

CRITICAL THINKING ACTIVITY

You are a nurse working in a physician's office. The physician prescribed Prednisone to a client for asthma. As you assess the client, she mentions that she is breast feeding. What action should you take?

CHAPTER 43

OVERVIEW OF THE RESPIRATORY SYSTEM

DEFINITION OF TERMS

Define the following:

1. airway resistance

2. apneustic center

3. alveolar ventilation

4. compliance

5. oxyhemoglobin

6. pneumotaxic

Match the terms in Column A with the appropriate phase in Column B

Column A		**Column B**
7. _____ Larynx	A.	membrane covering next to the lung
8. _____ Epiglottis	B.	tissue providing form for the nose
9. _____ Diaphragm	C.	primary muscle of inspiration
0. _____ Visceral pleura	D.	location of vocal cords
1. _____ Cartilage	E.	prevents aspiration of food into the lungs

Find the words that complete the statements below. They may appear diagonally, horizontall vertically, or backwards.

M	K	U	S	E	I	J	Y	O	P	Q	R	T	A	V	C
T	E	R	M	I	N	A	L	R	X	T	R	H	X	U	H
N	B	K	S	C	T	K	J	Y	N	A	B	I	D	I	B
A	Y	X	O	P	Q	L	M	X	C	A	S	M	G	T	K
T	G	N	K	M	W	R	B	H	C	F	E	H	R	H	U
C	A	Y	O	A	S	K	A	T	I	T	E	P	S	B	T
A	S	R	X	D	A	E	I	W	F	R	Q	L	E	G	A
F	A	A	Y	S	S	V	T	J	K	C	O	P	S	I	Y
R	W	L	G	Z	E	I	I	T	V	I	M	T	A	S	R
U	F	M	E	L	X	S	H	N	E	U	C	O	E	Z	O
S	E	C	N	A	T	S	I	S	E	R	Q	L	R	B	S
C	A	T	N	E	G	A	T	I	V	E	A	D	C	E	S
E	X	N	I	D	S	P	E	I	T	S	U	G	N	D	E
A	L	V	E	O	L	I	E	R	A	O	T	L	I	S	C
V	J	L	C	N	G	Y	R	A	L	L	I	P	A	C	C
D	E	C	R	E	A	S	E	D	N	U	R	S	E	I	A

12. Structures of the lower respiratory system begin after the _____.

13. The _____ is the largest airway in the body.

14. The _____ mainstem bronchus divides from the trachea in almost a straight line aspiration in this bronchus is common.

15. Mucociliary action is decreased by _____ _____.

16. The _____ respiratory unit is the principal site of gas exchange.

17. _____ reduces surface tension inside the alveoli.

18. Inspiration is an_____ process; whereas expiration is a_____ process.

19. Flow of inspired air is facilitated by the _____ pressure gradient.

20. With physical excursion, the _____ muscles are used to assist i expanding the thoracic cavity.

21. _____ is minimal in a large airway, but _____ as the airway becomes smaller.

22. _____ lung expansion can be an age-related change.

3. At the alveolar capillary, oxygen moves _____ the alveolus into the _____ blood.

4. Due to the _____ concentration of carbon dioxide in the capillary, carbon dioxide moves from the capillary into the _____.

5. Peripheral chemoreceptors are sensitive to the level of _____ in the blood.

CHAPTER 44

NASAL DECONGESTANTS, ANTITUSSIVES, AND MUCOLYTICS

DEFINITION OF TERMS

Complete the sentences, using the correct term for each definition.

allergic rhinitis, nasal congestion, dry and nonproductive cough, congested and nonproductive cough, rhinitis, congested and productive cough, sinusitis, common cold, rebound phenomenon, paradoxical reaction, and stomatitis

1. _____ is sneezing, runny nose, nasal itching, and nasal congestion.

2. _____ is mucous membrane engorgement resulting from dilation of the blood vessels in the nasal mucosa associated with rhinitis, allergic rhinitis, and colds.

3. _____ _____ is an unexpected or contradictory response to a drug.

4. A _____ and _____ cough produces a scant amount of sputum and is associated with chest congestion.

5. _____ is hypersensitivity reaction to inhaled antigens causing profuse watery nasal discharge, sneezing, swollen nasal mucosa, and itching of the nose and palate.

6. A _____ and _____ cough does not produce sputum and is not associated with chest congestion.

7. _____ _____ is the occurrence of extreme congestion of nasal passages when the decongestant's duration of action ends.

8. _____ , inflammation of a sinus cavity, produces fever, chills, nasal obstruction, and pain and tenderness of the involved sinus.

9. A _____ or coryza syndrome is a viral infectious process of the upper respiratory tract.

10. A _____ and _____ cough produces expectorated mucous and is associated with chest congestion.

11. _____ is erythema of the mucous membranes, dry mouth, and burning of the oral mucosa.

In the table below, identify the actions and uses of each type of drug

Type of Drug	Action	Uses
Nasal decongestants	12. Adrenergic drugs that shrink _____ of the nasal mucosa.	13. Relieve symptoms of colds, allergic rhinitis, sinusitis and adjunctive therapy in treating _____ _____ _____
Antihistamines	14. Block effect of _____ at receptor sites in the body.	Allergic rhinitis
Antitussives	15. Alleviate coughing by either depressing the cough center in the medulla or acting on receptors within the _____ _____.	16. Symptomatic relief of cough for either acute respiratory conditions or _____ _____.
Expectorants	17. Increase productivity of cough by stimulating the flow and reducing the _____ of respiratory tract secretions.	18. Symptomatic relief of respiratory conditions characterized by presence of _____ , _____ cough or mucous in respiratory tract.
Mucolytics	19. _____ secretions to make it easier to eliminate; may produce enhanced ciliary action. Soothes and cleanses mucous membranes.	20. Adjunctive treatment for abnormally _____ mucous secretions present with acute and chronic bronchopulmonary-pulmonary disease or pulmonary complications of cystic fibrosis.

For the client with severe allergic rhinitis, develop a nursing care plan containing three nursing diagnoses, goals, expected outcomes, and appropriate nursing interventions (See page 547 of text for suggestions.).

Nursing Diagnosis, Goal, and Expected Outcomes	Nursing Interventions
Nursing diagnosis #1: Goal: Expected Outcomes: Nursing diagnosis #2 Goal: Expected Outcomes: Nursing diagnosis #3 Goal: Expected Outcomes:	

MULTIPLE CHOICE

Select the best answer.

1. Which sentence best describes undesired clinical responses?
   A. A paradoxical reaction to nasal decongestants is restlessness, insomnia, euphoria, nervousness, and tremors.
   B. Stomatitis is an undesired reaction to expectorants.
   C. Chronic nasal congestion is an undesired reaction to nasal decongestants.
   D. Bronchospasm is an undesired reaction to peripherally acting antitussives.

2. Which choice is most appropriate regarding contraindications to these drugs?
   A. Nasal decongestants should be used with caution in clients with hypertension or cardiac disease.
   B. Expectorants should be used with caution in clients on monoamine oxidase inhibitor (MAOI) therapy.
   C. Peripherally acting antitussives should not be used with clients with bronchial asthma.
   D. Mucolytics should be avoided in clients with diabetes mellitus.

23. Which statement is most accurate about the histamine response?
   A. Histamine is responsible for the antiinflammatory response.
   B. Eosinophils contain large amounts of histamine.
   C. Histamine release results in decreased blood flow because of constricted capillaries.
   D. Histamine is released because of hypersensitivity reaction or tissue injury.

24. Which sentence best describes specific drug-related nursing considerations?
   A. Educate clients who are taking expectorants about the rebound phenomenon.
   B. Caution clients taking nasal decongestants about driving.
   C. Avoid the use of glass, stainless steel, and plastic with mucolytics.
   D. Encourage clients with mucous secretions to use water either orally or inhaled to eliminate secretions.

CRITICAL THINKING ACTIVITY

A friend who is in her first trimester of pregnancy asks you if she can take Neo-synephrine and Robitussin for a cold. What should you tell her?

CHAPTER 45
BRONCHODILATING DRUGS AND RELATED AGENTS

DEFINITION OF TERMS

Define the following:

1. bronchodilator

2. bronchopulmonary dysplasia

3. deoxyribonuclease

4. mast cell stabilizer

5. metered dose inhaler

BRONCHODILATOR PROTOTYPES

Complete the table. The hints in parentheses are words within the terms used to fill the blanks. The hint words may have the letters in different order than they appear in the term. The terms will be much longer than the hints.

Pharmacodynamics

Sympathomimetic Bronchodilator Prototype Albuterol	Methylxanthine Bronchodilator Prototype Theophylline
6. Selective B$_2$ (is) _____ 7. In inhaled form stimulates B$_2$ (pot) _____ located on bronchial smooth muscle, causing bronchodilation 8. May also stimulate B$_1$ receptors causing (card) _____	9. Bronchodilator and (sod) _____ 10. Increases cardiac output and heart rate, improves contractility of (rag) _____, accelerates (us) _____ transport by the cilia. Inhibits phosphodiesterase, dilating the bronchi

Contraindications and Precautions

Sympathomimetic Bronchodilator Prototype Albuterol	Methylxanthine Bronchodilator Prototype Theophylline
Hyperthyroidism 11. (on) _____ (art) _____ disease 12. (bat) _____ (us) _____ May inhibit uterine contractions and complicate labor and delivery Pregnancy category C drug	13. Upper (at) _____ tract infections in children slow clearance of drug and may result in toxicity Hypersensitivity 14. (tip) _____ (rule) _____ disease Seizure disorders Pregnancy Category C drug Present in breast milk, causing irritability in infants

Drug-Drug Interactions

Sympathomimetic Bronchodilator Prototype Albuterol	Methylxanthine Bronchodilator Prototype Theophylline
15. Use with other adrenergic aerosols may cause (radical) _____ (chap) _____ 16. ß-blockers (pose) _____ action 17. Sympathomimetic drugs have (dive) _____ effect	18. Smoking tobacco or marijuana (near) _____ drug clearance 19. Allopurinol, cimetidine, ciprofloxacin, erythromycin, oral (trace) _____, and rifampin

Compare and contrast undesired clinical responses to albuterol and theophylline for the following body systems.

20. Cardiac:

21. CNS:

22. GI:

23. Endocrine:

24. Integumentary:

ANTOCHOLINERGIC DRUG AND MAST CELL PROTOTYPES

Match the correct drug with the characteristic. You will have only one answer for each question. Use A to indicate ipratropium bromide (Atrovent) and B to indicate cromolyn sodium.

25. ____ Used to treat chronic bronchitis and emphysema

26. ____ Few drug-drug interactions

27. ____ Common undesired clinical responses are bronchospasm, cough, nasal congestion, throat irritation, and wheezing

28. ____ Dosage forms: inhaler or aerosol

29. ____ Used with caution in clients with impaired hepatic or renal function

30. ____ Used to treat mild to moderate asthma

31. ____ Antagonizes the action of acetylcholine, the neurotransmitter released from the vagus nerve

32. ____ Dosage forms: inhaler, nasal spray, nebulizer, and oral

33. ____ No bronchodilating action

34. ____ Adverse reactions are rare

35. ____ Common adverse reactions are nervousness, dizziness, headache, dry mouth, and cough

36. ____ Inhibits release of mediators after exposure to an antigen

37. ____ Should be used with caution in clients with glaucoma.

NURSING CONSIDERATIONS

Determine if each teaching statement is true or false. Correct the false statements.

38. ____ If you are on cromolyn you should increase fluid intake to increase the viscosity of lung secretions.

39. ____ Overuse of cromolyn may cause paradoxical bronchospasm.

40. ____ It is very important to store inhalation albuterol in a moist area with a constant temperature.

41. ____ While you are on theophylline it is important to eat a high-protein, low-carbohydrate diet because it increases the theophylline level.

42. ____ Avoid excessive use of caffeine, smoking, or second hand smoke while on albuterol.

43. ____ It is safe to increase the dose as needed of the albuterol inhaler but follow the dosage closely for the oral forms of this drug.

44. ____ Take theophylline with food or an antacid if GI symptoms occur, but food must be high fat.

45. ____ You should not exceed 6 inhalations of atrovent in 24 hours.

46. _____   Be careful not to spray atrovent into your eyes it will cause temporary blurred vision.

47. _____   Atrovent is not for occasional use, you must follow the dosage closely.

CRITICAL THINKING ACTIVITY

You are a nurse teaching a mother how to give nose drops to a toddler. The mother tells you that she thinks it is mean to hold the child down or restrain the child to put in the drops. What should you do?

Chapter 46
OVERVIEW OF THE DIGESTIVE SYSTEM

Definition of Terms

Match the term with the correct definition.

1. _____ accessory organs
2. _____ segmental contraction
3. _____ gastrointestinal tract
4. _____ adventitia
5. _____ propulsion
6. _____ tunics
7. _____ amylase
8. _____ brush border
9. _____ chyme
10. _____ microvilli
11. _____ rugae
12. _____ secretin
13. _____ villus

A. A semifluid material consisting of a mixture of food, fluid, and gastric secretions

B. The fourth layer of the GI tract consisting of connective tissue

C. Longitudinal folds of the tunica mucosa of the stomach that expand for stomach distention

D. An enzyme that begins the process of carbohydrate metabolism in the mouth

E. Ringlike contractions that mix and break up food

F. The microvilli of the small intestines

G. A fingerlike projection of the mucous membrane of the small intestine

H. The part of the digestive system beginning at the mouth and ending at the anus

I. The four layers that form the wall of the GI tract

J. Movement of food from one end of the tract to the other

K. Cytoplasmic extensions at the free surfaces of epithelial cells in the small intestine

L. Teeth, tongue, salivary glands, liver, gallbladder, and pancreas

M. A peptide hormone that stimulates the pancreas

FUNCTIONS OF THE GI TRACT

Complete the following sentences. The last letter of the correct word is provided for you.

Mouth

The soft palate serves as a partition between the (14.) _____ h and nasopharynx. It moves upward to close the nasopharyngeal opening during swallowing, preventing food and fluids from entering the (15.) _____ x.

Accessory Organs

The salivary glands produce (16.) _____ a, which contains mucus, serous secretions and amylase. Saliva (17.) _____ s food particles and serves as a (18.) _____ e shield for the mouth.

Teeth assist (19.) _____ n by cutting, tearing, grinding, and chewing food.

The tongue manipulates food, assists (20.) _____ g, determines sensation and taste, and cleanses teeth and gums.

Pharynx

The oropharynx and laryngopharynx transmit food from the mouth to the (21.) _____ s. The epiglottis closes the larynx while swallowing to prevent aspiration.

Esophagus

The vagus nerve stimulates contraction of muscles to open and close pharyngoesophageal and (22.) _____ l sphincters so they are open only during swallowing.

(23.) _____ c activity moves food through the esophagus to the stomach.

Stomach

The mucous coat (tunica mucosa) or innermost lining of the stomach contains the following types of cells:

The surface mucous or mucous neck cells secrete a (24.) _____ s that provides a protective coating for the stomach lining.

The (25.) _____ l cells produce hydrochloric acid and intrinsic factor. The hydrochloric acid activates (26.) _____ n, which initiates protein digestion. Intrinsic factor facilitates absorption of (27.) _____ n _____ in the small bowel.

The chief cells secrete (28.) _____ n, which forms pepsin when mixed with hydrochloric acid.

The endocrine cells secrete regulatory hormones that stimulate or inhibit (29.) _____ c secretion.

Small Intestine

The major organ for (30.) _____ n and absorption of nutrients.

The intestinal villi and the circular folds of the submucosal and mucosal coats create a large surface for (31.) _____ n.

Segmented contractions and peristaltic waves mix and churn the intestinal contents, moving the chyme against the (32.) _____ i. (33.) _____ s propels the chyme through the bowel.

The lining of the small intestine is protected by secretions from (34.) _____ 's gland in the duodenum, intestinal glands at the bases of the villi, and bicarbonate ions from th (35.) _____ s (stimulated by secretin from the duodenum).

Microvilli contain (36.) _____ e enzymes. Peptidase split peptides into amin acids; sucrase, maltase, and lactase split disaccharides into simple sugars; and intestina (37.) _____ e splits fats into fatty acids and glycerol.

Large Intestine

Major functions are absorption of water and (38.) _____ s from chyme remain ing in the alimentary canal and forming and storing feces until defecated.

Water, mucus, (39.) _____ m , and bicarbonate are secreted by cells in the larg intestine, stimulated by chyme and parasympathetic impulses. These substances (40.) _____ and protect the mucosa and help bind fecal matter together.

Mixing movements break fecal matter into segments and rotate to expose to intestinal mucosa and promote (41.) _____ n.

Mass movement, where a large segment of the intestinal wall constricts vigorously, forces th intestinal contents toward the (42.) _____ m. This stimulates the defecation reflex, which results in stimulation of peristalsis in the descending colon, involuntary relaxation of the (43.) _____ l anal sphincter, increased internal abdominal pressure, and volun tary relaxation of the external (44.) _____ r resulting in elimination of feces.

Liver

It has many important (45.) _____ c activities.

It plays a major role in (46.) _____ e metabolism by converting glucose t glycogen, glycogen to glucose, and noncarbohydrates to glucose. It is important to (47.) _____ metabolism to oxidize fatty acids and synthesize lipoproteins, phospholipids, and cholesterol. I protein metabolism, the liver forms (48.) _____ a, synthesizes blood proteins, and convert amino acids. It also assists in the storage of vitamins and minerals and (49.) _____ of harmful substances.

The liver secrets (50.) _____ e, which reduces the acidity of chyme, stimulates intestina motility, aids in utilization of protein and carbohydrates, emulsifies fat, increases lipase activity, an increases absorption of fat soluble vitamins (A, D, and K).

Gallbladder

It stores and concentrates (51.) _____ e between meals. Bile is released into the (52.) _____ m when the intestinal mucosa, stimulated by fat, secretes cholecysto kinin, which in turn, stimulates the gallbladder.

Pancreas

Secretes (53.) _____ e _____ e produced in the pancreatic acina cells. The juice is released into the pancreatic duct, which connects to the duodenum by the ampull of Vater.

Pancreatic juice contains (54.) _____ s that split carbohydrates, proteins, fats, an nucleic acids. Pancreatic juice also contains high (55.) _____ e ion concentration, which serves to neutralize chyme.

IMPACT OF DRUG THERAPY ON THE GI TRACT

56. List three types of drugs used on the upper GI tract:

57. List three conditions of the lower GI tract that might require drug therapy:

58. List three side effects and adverse reactions of the GI tract resulting from drug therapy.

MULTIPLE CHOICE

Select the best answer.

59. The total time that it takes food to travel the length of the GI tract is approximately:
    A. 6-8 hours.
    B. 10-12 hours.
    C. 24-36 hours.
    D. 48 hours.

60. The capacity of the stomach is:
    A. one milliliter.
    B. one-half liter.
    C. one liter.
    D. two liters.

61. Which statement is most accurate regarding gastric absorption and gastric emptying?
    A. The stomach wall is permeable to passage of most materials into the blood.
    B. The stomach absorbs water, glucose, electrolytes, certain drugs, and alcohol.
    C. Meals high in solids, fats, and protein empty quickly from the stomach.
    D. Tepid, isotonic liquids empty slowly from the stomach.

62. Which sentence best describes absorption in the small intestine?
    A. The jejunum is the only area for absorption of vitamin B_{12} complex and bile salts in the small intestine.
    B. The duodenum is the major part of the small intestine for nutrient absorption.
    C. The jejunum absorbs any nutrients not absorbed in the duodenum or ileum.
    D. Most fats are absorbed in the jejunum.

63. Which statement is most accurate concerning movements of the large intestine?
    A. Normal peristaltic waves occur almost continuously.
    B. The internal sphincter is under voluntary control.
    C. The mixing movements promote water and electrolyte absorption.
    D. The defecation reflex occurs as a result of feces being pushed into the descending colon.

CRITICAL THINKING ACTIVITY

If you wanted a drug that was taken with meals to absorb slowly, what type of meal would be best for the client to eat? Supply the rationale for your answer.

CHAPTER 47
DRUGS AFFECTING THE UPPER GASTROINTESTINAL TRACT

DEFINITION OF TERMS

Define the following:

1. acid neutralizing capacity

2. cephalic phase

3. dysphagia

4. eructation

5. flatulence

6. gastric phase

7. hypersecretion

8. hyposecretion

9. milk-alkali syndrome

10. proton pump

11. pyrosis

STUDY QUESTIONS

CASE STUDY

Ed Robensen, age 52, has been admitted to the ICU with bleeding ulcers. He is alert, anxious, and able to give a history. He complains of acute epigastric pain. He has a history of arthritis and takes aspirin or ibuprofen most days for pain. He works as a bank manager and describes his job as very stressful. He smokes 1 to 1 1/2 packs of cigarettes a day and drinks coffee all day long. He eats a varied diet and does not drink alcohol. He has no allergies.

The physician orders:
Nasogastric tube to low suction
IV 1000cc D5W alternated with 1000cc Lactated Ringers, infused 1000cc q 8 hours
Rantidine 50 mg IV infusion q 6 hours
CBC q a.m.
Maalox TC 10 ml q 2 hour by NG tube

12. What factors contributed to Mr. Robensen's ulcer condition?

13. List three nursing diagnoses for Mr. Robensen.

14. What are the expected effects of the rantidine (Zantac) and Maalox TC?

15. Prepare a discharge teaching plan for Mr. Robensen addressing diet and life-style.
Diet Modifications:

Life-style concerns:

Indicate if the statement is true or false. Correct the false statements.

5. _____ The three most common undesired clinical responses to cimetidine (Tagamet) are agitation, disorientation, and depression.

7. _____ The four groups of antisecretory drugs are H_2-receptor antagonists, antimuscarinic drugs, pump inhibitors, and prostaglandins.

3. _____ Concomitant administration of antacids is not recommended with many of the upper GI protective agents.

9. _____ It is important for omeprazole (Prilosec) to be taken with meals for optimal effect.

0. _____ Misoprostol (Cytotec) is classified as a Pregnancy Category C drug.

1. _____ Aluminum toxicity may occur with clients who have renal problems when taking either antacids with aluminum or antimuscarinics.

2. _____ Prothrombin time must be monitored carefully if the client is receiving both warfarin and either cimetidine (Tagamet) and omeprazole (Prilosec).

3. _____ It is considered safe to take antacids as needed with sucralfate (Carafate), as long as they are taken 30 minutes before or after the sucralfate.

4. _____ Administration of sucralfate (Carafate) concomitantly with other drugs produces few drug interactions.

5. _____ The most common side effects of antacids are diarrhea or constipation.

6. _____ Antacids are inorganic salts, combining a cation such as hydroxide, bicarbonate, citrate, carbonate, and phosphate with an anion such as magnesium, aluminum, sodium, and calcium.

7. _____ Helicobacter pylori infection increases gastric acid secretion and increases the risk for long-term ulcer recurrence.

8. _____ Some major antianxiety and antipsychotic agents, such as prochlorperazine, chlorpromazine, and thiethylperazine, are widely used as antiemetics.

Match the description with the most appropriate drug or drugs. There may be more tha one answer for each description (noted by plural s), but each answer is only used one time.

29. ____ Serotonin antagonist for emetogenic cancer therapy

30. ____ Used for acute poisoning

31. ____ Enzymes used for cystic fibrosis

32. ____ Antihistamines used for motion sickness

33. ____ Antidopaminergics used for severe nausea and vomiting

34. ____ Prostaglandin used for NSAID-induced gastric ulcers

35. ____ Used for gaseous distention

36. ____ Used for achlorhydria

37. ____ H₂ receptor antagonists for PUD, GERD, hypersecretion

38. ____ Pump inhibitor for duodenal ulcers, erosive esophagitis, hypersecretion

39. ____ Cytoprotective for short term treatment of gastric and duodenal ulcers

40. ____ Cannabinoid used for nausea and vomiting associated with cancer chemotherapy

A. misoprostol (Cytotec)

B. prochlorperazine (Compazine), metoclo ramide (Reglan)

C. omeprozole (Prilosec)

D. dronabinal (Marinol)

E. glutamic acid

F. odansetron (Zofran)

G. activated charcoal

H. promethazine (Phenergan), meclizir (Antivert, Bonine), dimenhydrinat (Dramamine)

I. pancrelipase (Cotazym, Protilase, Zymas

J. simethicone (Mylicon)

K. sucralfate (Carafate)

L. cimetidine (Tagamet), famotidine (Pepsi

MULTIPLE CHOICE

Select the best answer.

41. Omeprazole (prilosec) is not used for maintenance therapy for ulcer control because:
    A. it is too expensive.
    B. the duration of action is short.
    C. side effects are frequent and severe.
    D. gastric carcinogenic effects have been seen in animal studies.

42. A client receiving dronabinol (Marinol) ha developed psychoactive side effects. The in tial nursing action would be:
    A. contact the prescriber.
    B. withhold further drug treatment.
    C. provide a quiet environment with su pervision.
    D. request a serum drug level.

3. The client is receiving nizatidine (Axid) for maintenance control of duodenal ulcer. The client should be instructed to take the drug:
   A. before breakfast.
   B. one hour before the largest meal of the day.
   C. at bedtime.
   D. at the same time each day, preferably in the morning.

44. The least appropriate drug for a child with chemotherapy-induced nausea and vomiting would be:
   A. promethazine (Phenergan).
   B. chlorpromazine (Thorazine).
   C. ondansetron (Zofran).
   D. metoclopramide (Reglan).

CRITICAL THINKING ACTIVITY

A 78-year-old male client reports frequent acid-indigestion and heart-burn. He indicates that he has been taking "baking-soda water" to relieve the symptoms. What assessment data would be of most concern to the nurse?

Chapter 48
DRUGS AFFECTING THE LOWER GASTROINTESTINAL TRACT

Definition of Terms

Define the following:

1. cathartic

2. constipation

3. diarrhea

4. encopresis

5. hyperosmotic

6. lavage

7. laxative

8. osmotic

9. surfactant

NURSING INTERVENTIONS

State rationale for each of the nursing interventions.

Intervention	Rationale
Emphasize the need for excellent fluid intake for a client who is taking a bulk-forming laxative.	10.
Instruct client who is taking mineral oil to swallow the medication carefully and remain in an upright position for 2 hours afterward.	11.
Chill mineral oil before administering it, and offer the client fruit juice or other favorite beverage.	12.
Instruct the client who is taking oral bisacodyl (Dulcolax) that the tablets should not be crushed, chewed, or taken with milk.	13.
Assess a pediatric client with encopresis for constipation.	14.
Obtain information about current medication usage, including nonprescription drugs, from a client who complains of constipation.	15.
Instruct a client that a 1 gallon container of polyethylene glycol is to be taken in 3 to 4 hours (1 glass every 10 to 15 minutes)	16.
Assess vital signs, skin turgor, and oral mucous membranes in a client who complains of diarrhea.	17.

Interventions	Rationale
Before instructing a client on a bland/low residue diet for diarrhea, inquire about the client's tolerance of milk products.	18.
Advise a client who is taking Lomotil that it is best not to drive a car right after taking this medication.	19.
Inquire about history of glaucoma and/or enlarged prostate in an elderly client who is taking Lomotil.	20.
Encourage parents to check with their physician before giving Pepto-Bismol to a child with a fever and diarrhea.	21.
Encourage pregnant clients to maintain regular bowel elimination without drugs.	22.
Monitor the blood sugar carefully with a diabetic client who is on Sandostatin (octreotide acetate).	23.

MULTIPLE CHOICE

Select the best answer.

24. The risk of laxative dependency is greatest with habitual use of:
    - A. bulk-forming agents.
    - B. lubricants.
    - C. surfactants.
    - D. stimulants.

25. The rationale for adding atropine to Lomotil is to:
    - A. potentiate the action of diphenoxylate.
    - B. counteract the side effects of dipehoxylate.
    - C. discourage the abuse of Lomotil.
    - D. make the liquid form of Lomotil more palatable

26. Which statement is most accurate about Colace?
    - A. Chronic liver disease can occur with prolonged use.
    - B. It is considered habit forming.
    - C. It is used for functional constipation.
    - D. It decreases the absorption of digoxin and salicylates.

27. Which one of the following types of drugs may cause diarrhea?
    - A. anticholinergic drugs
    - B. antidepressants
    - C. cardiac glycosides
    - D. diuretics

28. The following nursing diagnoses have been identified in a client with diarrhea. Which one would be given priority?
    - A. Impaired skin integrity
    - B. Fluid volume deficit
    - C. Sleep pattern disturbance
    - D. Pain associated with cramping

Match the primary mechanism of action with the appropriate drug. Each answer is used only once.

LAXATIVES

29. _____ magnesium hydroxide suspension (Milk of Magnesia)

30. _____ bisacodyl (Dulcolax)

31. _____ psyllium hydrophilic colloid (Metamucil)

32. _____ polyethylene glycol solution (CoLyte, Golytely)

33. _____ docusate sodium (Colace)

34. _____ mineral oil

A. Emollient action allows water and fats to penetrate fecal mass

B. Draws additional water into the intestinal tract by osmosis

C. Washes out the lower intestinal tract with little gain or loss of body fluid

D. Stimulates sensory nerve endings in lining of intestinal mucosa

E. Lubricates the fecal mass and the lining of the bowel wall

F. Increases the fluid content and bulk of the stool

ANTIDIARRHEAL DRUGS

35. ____   activated attapulgite (Kaopectate)

36. ____   diphenoxylate with atropine (Lomotil)

37. ____   octreotide (Sandostatin)

38. ____   bismuth subsalicylate (Pepto-Bismol)

A.   Acts on central nervous system and depresses opioid receptors in intestinal wal

B.   Anti-inflammatory action inhibits GI secretion and motility

C.   Analogue of natural hormone, which ha potent antisecretory action

D.   Possible adsorbent of toxins in bowe (therapeutic action doubtful)

CRITICAL THINKING ACTIVITY

Eleanor C., a 70-year-old widow sought medical attention because of constipation and "feeling run down." Further history revealed that Eleanor had been experiencing fatigue, poor appetite, and an irregular pattern of bowel elimination for about 6 months. She was using various laxatives, particularly Milk of Magnesia and ExLax. Eleanor is taking antihypertensives for high blood pressure and NSAIDS for osteoarthritis.

What factors may have contributed to the constipation that Eleanor is experiencing?

What are the actions of the laxatives that Eleanor is taking?

What problems can occur with habitual use of these medications?

CHAPTER 49
OVERVIEW OF BIOLOGIC DEFENSE MECHANISMS

DEFINITION OF TERMS

Define the following:

1. active acquired immunity

2. allergen

3. antibody

4. antigen

5. chemotaxis

6. immunogen

7. interferon

8. lymphokines

9. margination

10. opsonization

11. pasive acquired immunity

12. reticuloendothelial system

NONSPECIFIC DEFENSE MECHANISMS

non-selectively directed against any foreign substances

External Nonspecific Defense Mechanisms
Give an example of each type of external barrier.

Anatomic barriers	Mechanical barriers	Chemical barriers	Microbic flora
(13.)	(14.)	(15.)	(16.)

Internal Nonspecific Defense Mechanisms

Blood cells	Phagocytosis	RES	Infalmmatory response	Interferons	Complement system	Opsonization

Fill in the blanks with the appropriate letters

Blood cells—Leukocytes

(17.) _ e _ t _ o-phils	Eosinophils	Basophils	(18.) _ _ _ _ cytes	Lymphocytes	Plasma cells

Phagocytosis

Neutrophils	(19.) _ a _ _ ophages	(20.) L _ m _ h _ k _ n _ s	Lysosomal enzymes
begin process	activated & moved	mediate macrophages	digest phagocytized particles

Reticuloendothelial System RES
Mononuclear phagocyte system

(21.) _ o _ _ le macrophages	Stationary macrophages
Travel in connective tissues or blood stream where needed	(22.) Reside in specific t _ _ _ _ _ — lymphoid tissue, spleen, liver, bone marrow, lungs and blood vessels

Inflammatory Response
Redness, swelling, heat, and pain

(23.) Hyperemia =increased _ l _ _ d flow	(24.) "Wall off" = fibrinogen _ _ _ _ s	Margination =attracts neutrophils	(25.) Endogenous pyrogens =circulate to hypothalamus-increases _ e _ p _ r _ t _ r _	
Edema =serous fluids & proteins	Chemotaxis =attracts neutrophils	Pus = by product		Leukocytosis = increased Leukocytes

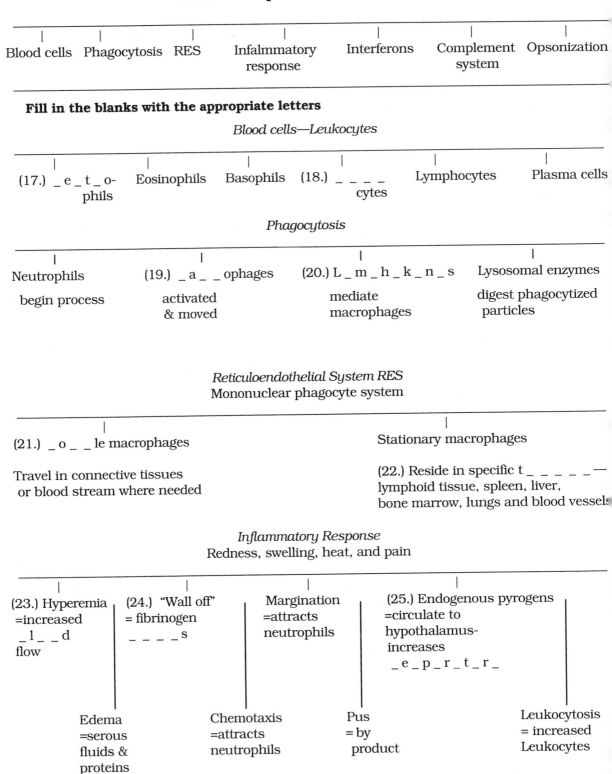

Interferons

(26.) _ _ _ e _ _ e _ cells release interferon which protects uninfected cells.

Complement System

Proteins	Pathways	Cascade reaction
(27.) 20 interacting _ l _ s _ a proteins Activation of enzyme precursors through pathways	Classic=IgM & IgG antibody/antigen response (28.) Alternate=IgA or _ i _ s _ e injury	(29.) Activated through _ a _ h _ a _ Products have enzymatic and biologic properties (30.)Various activities to e _ h _ n _ e immune response

Opsonization

(31.) Opsonin Elicited by _ n _ i _ _ d _ - _ n _ i _ e _ response and complement interactions	(32.) Antigens Coated and bound to _ ha _ _ c _ _ es

SPECIFIC DEFENSE MECHANISMS

Respond to specific foreign substances—the body's last line of defense.

Humoral-Mediated Immunity	Cell-Mediated Immunity

Humoral-Mediated Immunity
Short term—present in blood—remembers antigens and synthesizes antibodies

(33.) _ cells Respond to only one specific antigen (34.) May be transformed to plasma cells which can remember _ n _ i _ e _ s	Antibody Produced when B cells encounter specific antigen (35.) Fight antigen and activate _ o _ _ le _ e _ _ system	Immunoglobulins (36.) Chains of p _ _ y _ e _ t _ d _ s Some activate complement system

Cell-Mediated Immunity
Long term—present in lymph tissue—delayed sensitivity reactions

T lymphocytes or T cells

Helper cells

(37.) Major regulator of all

_ m _ _ _ e functions

Form lymphokines

Stimulate growth and
proliferation of effector and
suppressor cells

(38.) Stimulate B cells,
formation of plasma cells, and
secretion of _ n _ i _ o _ i _ s

Effector cells

(39.) Attack the

_ _ t _ _ e _ and
destroy through lysis

(40.) Suppressor cells

_ _ creases the immune
response to the antigen

(41.) Assists to differentiate

_ o _ e _ _ n from self

MULTIPLE CHOICE

Select the best answer.

42. Which statement is most accurate regarding
biologic defense mechanisms in the fetus
and newborn?
    A. By the third trimester, defense mecha-
nisms are mature in the fetus.
    B. Maternal transport of immunoglobu-
lins provides active protection for the
newborn the first few months of life.
    C. Most of the antibodies from the mother
are IgM.
    D. The newborn possesses a full number
of T cells, but they are not functional
until the fourteenth week after birth.

43. Which answer is correct about the effects ⌐
aging on biologic defense mechanisms?
    A. The main effects of aging are on th⌐
internal defense mechanisms.
    B. There is an increase in the number ⌐
anti-self antibodies.
    C. T-cells increase, B cells decrease.
    D. Cytotoxic activity decreases.

44. Which sentence best describes autoimmun⌐
diseases?
    A. They occur when there is an abnorma⌐
response of the immune system agains⌐
the body.
    B. They are always systemic diseases.
    C. They are caused by excessive huma⌐
leukocyte antigen (HLA) factors.
    D. They are caused when suppressor T⌐
cell activity is over stimulated.

CRITICAL THINKING ACTIVITY

You are taking care of a cancer patient who has a history of alcoholism. This patient
is receiving treatment with steroids and antineoplastic agents. What changes should
you be aware of in this client's immune system?

Chapter 50

HISTAMINE-RECEPTOR AGONISTS AND ANTAGONISTS

Definition of Terms

Define the following:

1. antigen

2. antihistamine

3. histamine

4. histamine antagonists

5. histamine-receptor antagonists

6. histamine-receptor blockers

Completion Exercise

7. Histamine is synthesized and stored in the _____ _____ and the _____.

8. Increased _____ _____ causes exudation of fluid and plasma proteins into the extravascular spaces and contributes to the formation of edema.

9. The H_1- receptor antagonists are more commonly referred to as _____ .

10. The _____ effect of many of the H_1- receptor antagonists produces symptoms of dry mouth and tenacious respiratory secretions.

11. Central nervous system _____ as a side effect of H_1-receptor therapy usually occurs in infants or children.

12. Prolonged use of topical preparations of H_1-receptor antagonists may result in a _____ reaction.

13. The second-generation H$_1$- receptor antagonists have a _____ onset of action than the first-generation drugs.

Study Questions

14. Identify contraindications to using H$_1$-receptor antagonists that have anticholinergic properties.

15. List undesired clinical responses to H$_1$-receptor antagonists that are more common in the elderly.

16. Describe the wheal-and-flare response. When would the nurse expect to see this response?

17. Prepare a chart that compares the antihistaminic, anticholinergic, and sedative properties of the prototype drugs for each of the sub-classes of H$_1$-receptor antagonists.

CRITICAL THINKING ACTIVITY

Explain the rationale for the following statements:

The use of H_1-receptor antagonists should be discontinued 4 days prior to skin testing for allergies.

The second-generation H_1- receptor antagonists are less likely to produce sedation than the first generation H_1- receptor antagonists.

Use of most of the H_1- receptor antagonists is contraindicated for clients with bronchial asthma.

CHAPTER 51
NONSTEROIDAL, ANTI-INFLAMMATORY DRUGS

DEFINITION OF TERMS

Define the following:

1. antipyretics

2. prostaglandin

3. Reye's syndrome

4. salicylate

5. salicylism

NONSTEROIDAL ANTI-INFLAMMATORY DRUGS

Complete the sentences.

The two groups of NSAIDS are (6.)_____ _____
_____ (_____) and (7.)_____
_____ _____ (_____).

The three major therapeutic uses for NSAIDS are: (8.)_____ (9.)_____
(10.)_____.

PSIs act primarily to prevent (11.)_____ and (12.)_____ of prostaglandins.

rostaglandins are synthesized and released when there is (13.) _____ to a cell membrane.

ome prostaglandins (PGE2) may contribute to the pathology associated with (14.) _____

_____ _____.

on-PSIs are either weak (15.) _____ or produce their effects by (16.) _____

_____.

SI-DRUG INTERACTIONS

Complete the possible reactions for drugs that interact with PSIs.

Interacting drug	Possible Reaction
Anticoagulants	17.
Antihypertensive drugs	18.
Diuretics	19.
Lithium	20.
Methotrexate	21.
Other PSIs	22.
Alcohol	23.

PROTOTYPE PSIs

Insert the missing letters or numbers.

Pharmacotherapeutics

Acetylsalicylic Acid (Aspirin)	Acetic Acid Derivative (indomethacin—Indocin)	Propionic Acid Derivative (ibuprofen—Motrin, Advil, Nuprin)
Wide variety of inflammatory disorders such as rheumatic arthritis and osteoarthritis, fever, headache, myalgias, dysmenorrhea, prevention of (24.) _ _ _ d _ o - _ _ s _ u _ a _ disorders	Osteoarthritis, ankylosing spondylitis, and rheumatoid (25.) _ _ _ h _ _ t _ _ , acute gouty arthritis, acute bursitis, and acute tendinitis. Also used to close patent ductus arteriosus in premature infants	Anti-inflammatory, mild antispasmodic, and antipyretic Rheumatoid arthritis, osteoarthritis, relief of musculoskeletal pain, (26.) d _ s _ e_ o _ _ _ e_

Pharmacokinetics

Acetylsalicylic Acid (Aspirin)	Acetic Acid Derivative (indomethacin—Indocin)	Propionic Acid Derivative (ibuprofen—Motrin, Advil, Nuprin)
Absorbed rapidly and completely in stomach and small intestine Bound to albumin Peak levels in (27.) ___ to ___ hours from oral administration Biotransformation in liver Metabolites excreted in urine (28.) Half-life: low dose= ___ to ___ hours large dose= 9-16 hours increased in elderly	Rapidly absorbed from the (29.) _ _ _ r _ c _ , including rectal mucosa for suppositories Bound to (30.) p _ a_ _ a _ r _ t _ i _ s Peak plasma levels in 2 hours Metabolized in liver Excreted in urine and (31.) _ _ l _ as unchanged compound and metabolites Distributed to all body fluids and tissues Half life of 4-5 hours	Well absorbed in GI tract Peak effect 1-2 hours Metabolized in (32.) _ _ _ e _ Excreted by (33.) _ i _ _ e _ _ Half-life=2 to 2 1/2 hours Excretion complete within (34.) _ _ hours of last dose Displaces other drugs bound to plasma protein

Pharmacodynamics

Acetylsalicylic Acid (Aspirin)	Acetic Acid Derivative (indomethacin—Indocin)	Propionic Acid Derivative (ibuprofen—Motrin, Advil, Nuprin)
(35.) Inhibits _ _ _ _ n _ _ e s _ _ Inhibits thromboxane A2 and prolongs bleeding time Systemic effect	Actions of aspirin, inhibits PG synthesis (36.) ___ to ___ times more potent than aspirin Decreases production of renin in kidney	Inhibits PG synthesis (37.) Reduces PG levels in _ e_ _ _ r _ a _ fluid and inhibits u _ _ _ _ _ _ contractions

STUDY QUESTIONS

38. List four miscellaneous PSIs. Compare these drugs with acetylsalicylic acid and propionic acid derivatives.

39. List three types of non-PSIs. Describe the pharmacodynamic properties of each.

40. Describe undesired clinical responses associated with gold salts.

41. List specific drug-related nursing interventions for the client receiving gold salts.

MULTIPLE CHOICE

Select the best answer.

42. Which statement is most accurate about undesired responses to PSIs?
    A. GI symptoms are caused by increased intestinal motility.
    B. Reproduction is influenced because of the effect on gonadotrophic hormones.
    C. Kidney function is affected by interference with normal prostaglandin functions.
    D. Hypersensitivity reactions are caused by stimulation of the adrenal glands.

43. Which sentence best describes nonprostaglandin synthetase inhibitors?
    A. Acetaminophen is as effective an anti-inflammatory agent as PSIs.
    B. Hyperuricemic drugs are used to treat gout.
    C. Gold salts are used to treat most forms of arthritis.
    D. Gold therapy has a few mild undesired side effects.

CRITICAL THINKING ACTIVITY

Which undesired clinical system responses common to PSIs has the potential to be the most harmful?

CHAPTER 52
IMMUNOSUPPRESSANT AND IMMUNOSTIMULANT DRUGS

DEFINITION OF TERMS

Match the term with the correct definition.

1. _____ Autoimmune diseases

2. _____ Cycle-specific drugs

3. _____ Immunostimulants

4. _____ Immunosuppressants

5. _____ Isoimmune reaction

6. _____ Phase-specific drugs

7. _____ Active immunity

8. _____ Passive immunity

9. _____ Toxoid

10. _____ Vaccine

A. Drugs that act on cells during a specific phase of the mitotic cycle

B. A suspension of live attenuated or killed microorganisms.

C. An immunologic response by the immune system of one individual against tissues of another individual.

D. Drugs that act on cells at all stages of the mitotic cycle.

E. Immunity that is conferred through administration of antibodies or sensitized lymphocytes produced by another individual or animal.

F. Drugs that suppress or inhibit the action of the immune system.

G. A bacterial toxin that has been treated with heat or a chemical agent to destroy its toxic properties without destroying its antigenic qualities.

H. Conditions that occur when components of the immune system are unable to differentiate self from foreign materials.

I. Immunity produced when immune bodies are actively formed by the host against specific antigens.

J. Drugs that stimulate the response of the immune system to specific antigens.

Unscramble the words to list the four categories of immunosuppressant drugs.

Categories of Immunosuppressant Drugs

11. Notixotcys	12. Peleh-Tr lecl	13. Tychlyemop	14. Doresitocsitroc
_____	Pusosreprss	Ditenobais	_____
	_____	_____	
	_____	_____	
	_____		

NURSING CONSIDERATIONS

Develop a nursing care plan for a patient on immunosuppressant therapy, using the following diagnosis: "High risk for infection related/to suppressed immune response." Develop three expected outcomes and appropriate interventions for each. Your evaluation would then be on outcome attainment. List specific areas of teaching under interventions.

Nursing Diagnosis: High risk for infection related to suppressed immune response.

Client-centered outcomes	Interventions
Goal: Client will remain free of serious infection while on immunosuppressant therapy. Expected outcome Expected outcome Expected outcome	

PROTOTYPES OF IMMUNOSUPPRESSANT DRUGS

Fill in the blanks.

Pharmacotherapeutics

Cytotoxic Immunosuppressant azathioprine (Imuran)	T-Helper Cell Suppressor cyclosporine (Sandimmune)
Prevention of transplant rejection, primarily (15.) _____ homotransplantation Treatment of severe rheumatoid arthritis resistant to conventional therapy	Prevention of rejection of solid organ transplants--kidney, liver, pancreas, and heart Prevention of problems with (16.) _____ _____ _____ Autoimmune disorders (Not used for chronic transplant rejection)

Pharmacokinetics

Cytotoxic Immunosuppressant azathioprine (Imuran)	T-Helper Cell Suppressor cyclosporine (Sandimmune)
Well absorbed after oral administration Peak levels (17.) ____ – ____ hours (oral administration) Bioavailability 41–44% (18.) _____ than IV administration Half-life ¹/₂ to 1 hour Rapidly converted to 6-mercaptopurine and other active metabolites Bound to serum proteins Oxidized or methylated in the (19.) _____ and liver Metabolites excreted by kidneys Most of drug and metabolites are no longer present in (20.) _____ after 8 hours	Oral form absorbed primarily in (21.) _____ _____ —slow, variable and incomplete Oral bioavailability is 30% Highly bound to erythrocytes and (22.) _____ _____ Blood distribution depends on drug concentration, hematocrit level, and lipoprotein concentration Lipid soluble so distributed throughout body to (23.) _____ and _____ cells Peak blood level 1-8 hours (oral administration) Extensive metabolism by liver enzymes. Half-life 7 hours for children, (24.) ____ hours for adults Major elimination route is (25.) _____, very little in (26.) _____

Pharmacodynamics

Cytotoxic Immunosuppressant azathioprine (Imuran)	T-Helper Cell Suppressor cyclosporine (Sandimmune)
Kill cells capable of (27.)_____ - _____ Acts by suppressing both (28.)_____ and _____ synthesis during initial stages of lymphoid cell differentiation Decreases initial proliferation and maturation of both T and B lymphocytes in response to (29.)_____ antigen Greater immunosuppressive effects for (30.)_____ -mediated immunity, rather than antibody-mediated immunity, so it works for prevention of transplant rejection rather than treatment Mechanism for arthritis not understood, except that it inhibits prostaglandin production and local inflammatory reactions	Does NOT cause generalized suppression of (31.)_____ _____cell production Selectively suppresses activation of (32.)___ - _____ cells by blocking synthesis and secretion of interleukin-2 Impairs cell-mediated response without destroying effector lymphocyte Does not prevent immune cells already activated by an antigen from (33.)_____ and differentiating

Undesired Clinical Responses

Cytotoxic Immunosuppressant azathioprine (Imuran)	T-Helper Cell Suppressor cyclosporine (Sandimmune)
Increased risk with (34.)_____ doses to prevent transplant rejection Most frequent effects are (35.)_____ and (36.)_____ . Causes (37.)_____ with leukopenia and thrombocytopenia. Also may cause macrocytic anemia, pure red cell aplasias, and reticulocytopenia. Myelosuppression is reversible with decreased or discontinued dosage. GI effects are most often (38.)_____ and _____ . Also diarrhea, fever, malaise, abdominal pain, constipation, anorexia mucositis, and hepatotoxicity Predisposition to (39.)_____ , renal insufficiency, and alopecia	Acute or chronic (40.)_____ _____ almost universal response. Dose dependent and generally reversible Reversible (41.)_____ common Hypertension, hyperglycemia, extremity tremor, anxiety, insomnia, gingival hyperplasia, sensory paresthesia, hirsutism, salt retention, hyperkalemia, hyperuricemia, hypomagnesemia, and fluid retention

Specific Drug-Related Nursing Considerations

Cytotoxic Immunosuppressant azathioprine (Imuran)	T-Helper Cell Suppressor cyclosporine (Sandimmune)
Pregnancy Category D drug (42.) _____ _____ for pregnant women Not recommended for (43.) _____ _____ Avoid (44.) _____ _____ with solution	(45.) _____ at therapeutic concentrations Monitoring (46.) _____ _____ important—consistency of measurement techniques and sample source Assess for drug toxicity or undesired clinical responses—especially (47.) _____ and _____ Instruct client in (48.) _____ hygiene Work with client to cope with hirsutism Pregnancy Category C drug Not recommended for breast feeding mothers Children prone to (49.) _____ drug levels

PROTOTYPES OF ANTIBODIES

Pharmacotherapeutics

Polyclonal Antibodies lymphocyte immune globulin (Atgam)	Monoclonal Antibodies muromonab-CD3 (Orthoclone OKT3)
Treatment of (50.) _____ rejection associated with renal transplantation (51.) _____ anemia Administered concurrently with other immunosuppressant drugs	(52.) _____ transplant rejection

Pharmacodynamics

Polyclonal Antibody lymphocyte immune globulin (Atgam)	Monoclonal Antibodies muromonab-CD3 (Orthoclone OKT3)
Impairs (53.) _____ - _____ responses by altering the function of T lymphocytes	Action specific to lymphocyte membrane (54.) _____ Binds to CD3 receptors found only on mature circulating T cells and medullary thymocytes. Blocks ability of cells to recognize (55.) _____ _____, inhibiting the generation and function of cytotoxic .T cells responsible for graft rejection

Undesired Clinical Responses

Polyclonal Antibody lymphocyte immune globulin (Atgam)	Monoclonal Antibodies muromonab-CD3 (Orthoclone OKT3)
(56.) _____, chills, fever, itching, erythema, and hemolysis (57.) _____ phlebitis	Majority of clients experience mild-to-severe (58.)" ____ - _____ " symptoms with first doses: fever, chills, headache, nausea, vomiting, diarrhea, and malaise. May decrease with subsequent injections Less frequent: marked hypotension, aseptic meningitis, acute decline in (59.) _____ _____ _____

Nursing Considerations

Polyclonal Antibody lymphocyte immune globulin (Atgam)	Monoclonal Antibodies muromonab-CD3 (Orthoclone OKT3)
(60.) _____ - _____ before first infusion (61.) _____ and emergency equipment available Administer through (62.) _____ - _____ vein	May be premedicated with antihistamines, acetaminophen, and (63.) _____

MULTIPLE CHOICE

Select the best answer.

64. Which statement is most accurate about general characteristics of immunosuppressant drugs?
    A. Most immunosuppressant drugs inhibit only one specific immune response.
    B. All available immunosuppressant drugs are highly toxic.
    C. Cytotoxins are the most commonly used immunosuppressant drugs.
    D. Corticosteroids are the only immunosuppressant drugs that produce generalized immune suppression.

65. Which choice is most appropriate about drugs producing passive immunity?
    A. Drugs used to impart passive immunity are used to treat exposure to an antigen, rather than as a prophylactic before exposure.
    B. Drugs producing passive immunity are contraindicated during pregnancy unless specifically needed.
    C. Live virus vaccinations may be given weeks after receiving immune globulin.
    D. Allergic reaction is more likely to occur with vaccinations producing active immunity.

66. Which answer about Rh (D) Immune Globulin is correct?
    A. It is effective for up to 72 hours after delivery in preventing maternal sensitization to Rh antigens.
    B. It is used to suppress the immune response of sensitized Rh (D) negative individuals who are exposed to Rh (D) positive blood.
    C. It is usually used during pregnancy.
    D. It is used for mothers who have Rh (D) negative fetuses.

67. Nurses who are giving immunostimulant drugs should consider that:
    A. Immunosuppressed clients should get killed vaccines only.
    B. Vaccines may be given to pregnant and nursing women, unless allergic to feathers or thimerosal.
    C. Live vaccines should not be administered concurrently but must be given 6-8 weeks apart.
    D. Live vaccines are shed in the stool and pharyngeal secretions for 6-8 weeks after immunization.

68. Which statement is most accurate about contraindications and side effects of immunostimulants producing active immunity?
    A. Symptoms of fever, fretfulness, anorexia, and vomiting following immunization are contraindications to further immunization with that agent.
    B. Undesired clinical responses to immunizations include anaphylaxis, convulsions, encephalopathy, encephalitis, and optic neuritis.
    C. Allergies are not a contraindication to immunization unless they include chickens, feathers, or eggs.
    D. Erythema at the injection site is usually an indication of hypersensitivity to the vaccine.

CRITICAL THINKING ACTIVITY

Which choice is most appropriate about nursing care of client on cytotoxic immunosuppressant drugs?
A. The nurse should hold the dose and notify the primary care provider if WBC>5000/mm.
B. The nurse should observe for signs of thrombocytopenia such as jaundice and elevated liver enzymes and bilirubin.
C. The nurse should hold the dose and consult the physician if the platelet count <20,000/mm.
D. The nurse should observe for signs of anemia such as epistaxis and hemoptysis.

Explain the rationale for your choice.

CHAPTER 53
HIV THERAPY

DEFINITION OF TERMS

Complete the sentences, choosing the correct term for each definition.

Acquired immunodeficiency syndrome, human immunodeficiency virus, retrovirus, macrolides, an opportunistic infections.

1. Broad spectrum antibiotics that act by inhibiting bacterial protein synthesis are _____

2. A virus containing RNA and reverse transcriptase that primarily infects CD4+ T-helper cells is _____.

3. The virus that causes progressive deterioration in cell-mediated immunity is th _____.

4. Infections caused by microorganisms that are ordinarily non-virulent and do not cause diseas are _____ .

5. A disease resulting in dysfunction of the immune system is _____.

DRUGS THAT INHIBIT REPLICATION OF HIV

HIV REPLICATION PROHIBITOR PROTOTYPE: ZIDOVUDINE (AZT, RETROVIR)

Complete the tables.

Pharmacokinetics
Absorption: (6.) _____
Peak serum concentrations: (7.) _____
Serum half-life: (8.) _____
Crosses (9.) _____ . _____ barriers.
Metabolized: (10.) _____, excreted: (11.) _____
Oral dose bioavailability is 65%

Pharmacodynamics

Inhibits: (12.) _____

Cellular thymidine kinase converts zidovudine into zidovudine (13.) _____

which is further converted to a (14.) _____ derivative, the active form.

Undesired Clinical Responses

(15.) _____ which decrease after 3–4 weeks of treatment.

(16.) _____ is common with high doses.

Neutropenia and thrombocytopenia due to (17.) _____ suppression

(18.) _____ of the proximal muscles of legs or arms

Contraindications and Precautions

(19.) Impaired _____ function

NURSING CONSIDERATIONS

Develop a nursing care plan for a client receiving drugs for HIV or AIDS, using the nursing diagnosis "High risk for altered health maintenance related to lack of knowledge of etiology and transmission of the disease, clinical course, and treatment plan." Develop three expected outcomes and interventions.

Expected Outcomes	Interventions
Expected Outcome	
Expected Outcome	
Expected Outcome	

MULTIPLE CHOICE

Select the best answer.

20. Which statement is most accurate about drug-drug interactions with zidovudine?
    A.   Ganciclovir is given concurrently to prevent bone marrow suppression.
    B.   Didanosine is only used concurrently with zidovudine.
    C.   Any drug having an adverse effect on renal function is contraindicated.
    D.   Probenecid caused hepatotoxicity when used with zidovudine.

21. Teaching for a client on zidovudine should include which of the following?
    A.   report any signs of nausea, vomiting, or abdominal pain.
    B.   Breast feeding is permitted while on drug therapy.
    C.   Always take the drug with meals.

22. Which answer is correct concerning drug that inhibit replication of HIV?
    A.   All of these drugs inhibit the revers transcriptase of HIV.
    B.   Excessive amounts of recombinar soluble CD4 is given to bind to the HI geome.
    C.   The most serious toxicity with zalcita bine is pancreatitis.
    D.   Peripheral neuropathy may occur wit both didanosine or zalcitabine.

CRITICAL THINKING ACTIVITY

You are caring for an HIV positive client who asks if he can continue drinking a cocktail every night with dinner. How should you respond?

CHAPTER 54
PRINCIPLES OF ANTIMICROBIAL THERAPY

DEFINITION OF TERMS

Unscramble the term that fits the definition.

1. A location where microorganisms can multiply. Sirerorev _____

2. The number and type of organisms vulnerable to the effects of an antimicrobial drug.
   Murtceps fo citativy _____ ____ _____

3. An invasion by and multiplication of an organism in body tissues. Tofinenic _____

4. The interval from onset of nonspecific clinical manifestations to more specific ones.
   Ramolodrp gates _____ _____

5. Drugs that affect a relatively limited number of microorganisms. Raworn tepurcms _____
   _____

6. The interval between the entrance of the pathogenic organism into the body and the appearance
   of the first symptoms. Nabocinuti doperi _____ _____

7. Organisms that exist in the presence of oxygen. Bericao _____

8. Drugs that affect a wide range of organisms. Roadb recutsmp _____ _____

9. The degree of resistance or immunity to pathogens. Ytilibitpecsus _____

0. An infectious agent including bacteria, viruses, fungi, and protozoa that cause disease.
   Gohenatp _____

1. Organisms that cannot exist in the presence of oxygen. Rincobea _____

2. A very small organism such as a bacteria or virus that can only be seen with the aid of a
   microscope. Nogomcarsimir _____

COMPLETION EXERCISE

Complete the following table on drugs classified by mechanism of action.

Mechanism of Action			
Mechanism	**Action**	**Result**	**Example**
Inhibition of cell wall synthesis	Affects (13.) _____ necessary for cell wall formation and integrity Bactericidal	(14.) _____ of cell and destruction of organism	(15.) _____
Inhibition of protein synthesis	Formation of (16.) _____ proteins Bind to cellular (17.) _____ Bactericidal or Bacteriostatic	Impedance of translation of (18.) _____ material Prevent (19.) _____ of genetic material and reproduction	Aminoglycosides and (20.) _____
Alteration of cell wall permeability	(21.) _____ to specific cell wall components	Alters (22.) _____ of cell wall, resulting in leakage of intracellular components	Amphotericin B
Inhibition of cellular metabolic processes	Block or alter (23.) _____ pathways	Suppress normal functioning of (24.) _____	(25.) _____
Inhibition of nucleic acid synthesis	Inhibit (26.) _____ and _____ synthesis	Restrict normal functioning of cell	(27.) _____ drugs

SELECTION OF ANTIMICROBIAL DRUGS

List two factors to consider for each of the following when selecting antimicrobial drugs.

28. Infecting pathogen _____

_____

29. Site of infection _____

_____

30. The client or recipient of the drug _____

_____

UNDESIRED RESPONSES TO ANTIMICROBIALS

Match the type of reaction with the appropriate description. You will have two answers for each reaction.

31. ___ ___   allergies and hypersensitivities

32. ___ ___   superinfections

33. ___ ___   organ toxicity

34. ___ ___   gastrointestinal effects

A.   Can result in blood dyscrasias and aplastic anemias

B.   Occurs often with oral or combination therapy

C.   From the suppression or destruction of normal flora

D.   Symptoms are diarrhea, nausea, vomiting, and abdominal discomfort

E.   Range from skin rashes to anaphylactic shock and death

F.   Results in overgrowth of pathogenic organisms

G.   May involve teeth, nail, and bones

H.   Can occur from either indirect or direct exposure

MULTIPLE CHOICE

Select the best answer.

35. Which statement is most accurate about spectrum of activity of antimicrobial drugs?
    A.   Drugs classified as aerobic and anaerobic refer to their activity levels.
    B.   The most common laboratory staining procedure to differentiate drugs is the Gram stain.
    C.   Broad spectrum drugs are less likely to destroy normal flora.
    D.   Narrow spectrum drugs are usually used to treat infections of unknown origin.

36. Which answer is correct regarding acquired resistance to antimicrobials?
    A.   Resistant strains of Staphylococcus aureus are common causes of nosocomial (hospital) infections.
    B.   The first emergence of drug resistant organisms was penicillin-resistant streptococcus.
    C.   The wide-spread use of narrow spectrum antibiotics such as penicillins contributed to the emergence of drug-resistant organisms.
    D.   Cross-resistance to other drugs of similar chemical composition is rare.

37. Which sentence best describes undesired responses to antimicrobials?
    A. Narrow spectrum antibiotics are more likely to produce GI problems.
    B. Sensitivity is usually specific with one drug and does not occur across related microbials.
    C. Antibiotics that are used to treat cancer are the only antimicrobials that are toxic to organs.
    D. Allergic and hypersensitive reactions are the most common responses to antimicrobials.

CRITICAL THINKING ACTIVITY

For each link in the chain of infection, describe a nursing intervention that could break the infection chain.

CHAPTER 55
ANTIBIOTICS

DEFINITION OF TERMS

Define the following:

1. crystalluria

2. kernicterus

3. nephrotoxicity

4. ototoxicity

5. pseudolithiasis

6. pseudomembranous colitis

7. ß-lactam

8. ß-lactamase

MECHANISMS OF ACTION FOR ANTIBIOTICS

Match the drug group with the mechanism of action. You will use some of the mechanisms for more than one drug group.

9. ____ Penicillin

10. ____ Cephalosporins

11. ____ Aminoglycosides

12. ____ Quinolones

13. ____ Macrolides

14. ____ Sulfonamides

15. ____ Tetracyclines

16. ____ Clindamycin

17. ____ Chloramphenicol

18. ____ Vancomycin

19. ____ Imipenem-Cliastatin

A.   Inhibits protein synthesis

B.   Interferes intracellularly by binding to sub units of bacterial ribosomes

C.   Interferes intracellularly by inhibiting DNA gyrase

D.   Inhibits bacterial cell wall synthesis

E.   Inhibits bacterial peptide bond formation and subsequent protein synthesis

F.   Prevents folic acid synthesis

G.   Interferes intracellularly by irreversibl binding to the subunit of the ribosoma ring

QUINOLONES AND MACROLIDES

Match the correct drug group with the characteristic.

A. Quinolones   B. Macrolides

20. ____ Includes ciprofloxacin (Cipro), norfloxacin, ofloxacin

21. ____ Drug-drug interactions include theophylline, aminophylline, antacids, and warfarin

22. ____ Undesired clinical responses are frequent GI problems, hypersensitivity, oral candidiasis and cholestatic jaundice

23. ____ Precautions are for pregnancy, breast feeding, children up to 18 years, CNS disorder and impaired renal function

24. ____ Drug-drug interactions are: carbamazepine, warfarin, cyclosporine, hepatotoxic drugs and theophylline

25. ____ Precautions are for impaired liver function

26. ____ Undesired clinical responses are GI upsets and CNS dizziness or lightheadedness headache, nervousness, drowsiness, or insomnia

27. ____ Include erythromycin and clarithromycin

UNDESIRED CLINICAL RESPONSES

For each undesired clinical response, identify the antibiotic(s) involved.
S=sulfonamides T=tetracyclines CH=chloramphenicol CL=clindamycin V=vancomycin
You may have more than one antibiotic for each undesired clinical response.

8. _____ Allergic (hypersensitivity) skin reactions such as rashes

9. _____ Liver toxicity, necrosis, or increase in liver enzymes

0. _____ Photosensitivity

1. _____ Optic neuritis

2. _____ Severe colitis

3. _____ Crystalluria

4. _____ GI upsets

5. _____ Nephrotoxicity

6. _____ Serious and fatal blood dyscrasias

7. _____ Moderate blood dyscrasias

8. _____ Permanent brown discoloration of teeth in children

9. _____ Ototoxicity

0. _____ Drug fever

1. _____ Peripheral neuritis

NURSING CONSIDERATIONS

Indicate if the statement is true or false. Correct the false statements.

2. _____ Clients taking ciprofloxacin should avoid sunlight or ultraviolet exposure and wear sunscreen and protective clothing to prevent a hypersensitivity reaction.

3. _____ Clients who are taking Cipro and antacids should take antacids 2-4 hours before or after the Cipro.

4. _____ Clients allergic to penicillin should not receive cephalosporins.

5. _____ Gray syndrome is an undesired clinical response to Bactrim that consists of aching joints and muscles, redness, blistering, peeling of skin, and unusual tiredness or weakness.

6. _____ Alcohol should not be taken with Cleocin because of resulting skeletal muscle weakness and respiratory depression.

7. _____ Clients taking erythromycin should be alert for signs such as dark or amber urine, pale stools, stomach pain, unusual tiredness, weakness, and jaundiced skin or eyes, which may indicate nephrotoxicity.

8. _____ Estrogen-containing oral contraceptives given concurrently with long-term tetracycline therapy may reduce contraceptive reliability and increase breakthrough bleeding.

49. ____   The most common drug allergy is to sulfonamides.

50. ____   Vancomycin IV should be infused over 30 minutes to prevent too rapid infusion of th drug resulting in "red-man" or "red-neck" syndrome.

Complete the rationale for the following nursing-teaching interventions.

Nursing-Teaching Interventions	Rationale
Instruct clients taking ciprofloxacin to take the oral drug with a full glass of water and drink several glasses of water between meals.	51.
Instruct clients taking erythromycin or Septra to take it with 240 mL of water 1 hour before or 2 hours after food or beverages.	52.
Instruct clients not to take sulfonamides if they are breast feeding.	53.
Instruct clients not to eat dairy products or antacids concurrently with some tetracyclines.	54.
Avoid tetracyclines during pregnancy and with children under 8 years.	55.
Chloramphenicol should not be taken by pregnant women at term (or during labor)	56.

MULTIPLE CHOICE

Select the best answer.

57. Which choice reflects correct administration of penicillin by the nurse?
   A. Natural penicillin and methicillin should be administered by shallow IM injection.
   B. Penicillin G and Staphcillin should be given orally 30 minutes before or 2 hours after meals.
   C. Penicillin G and Ampicillin are only given orally.
   D. Food increases absorption of ticarcillin, so it should be given with meals.

58. Which drug-drug interactions should th nurse be aware of when giving penicillin?
   A. Penicillin G may cause elevated sodiu levels when given with angiotensir converting enzyme inhibitors.
   B. Ticar should not be given with penici linase-resistant penicillins because the danger of blood dyscrasias.
   C. Methicillin should not be given wit other nephrotoxic drugs because of th possibility of interstitial nephritis.
   D. Ampicillin potentiates the effectivenes of estrogen-containing oral contracep tives.

59. Which contraindications and precautions should the nurse consider before giving penicillin?
    A. Staphcillin should be given with caution for clients on sodium restriction.
    B. Ticar should be given with caution to clients with mononucleosis.
    C. Ampicillin should be given with caution to clients with urinary tract infections.
    D. Penicillin G should be used with caution in clients with rheumatic fever.

60. Which statement is most accurate about penicillin-related drugs?
    A. Carbenicillin (Geocillin) is a B-lactam antibiotic used to treat bone and joint infections.
    B. Imipenem (Primaxin is a B-lactam antibiotic that is contraindicated with CNS or renal disorders.
    C. Mezlocillin (Mezlin) and aztreonam are used with aminoglycosides for synergistic effects against some microorganisms.
    D. Piperacillin (Pipracil) is a narrow spectrum antibiotic active only against aerobic, gram-negative organisms.

61. Which answer is correct about the generations of cephalosporins?
    A. First generation cephalosporins are most effective against methicillin-resistant gram-positive cocci.
    B. Second generation cephalosporins are most effective against both gram-positive and negative bacilli.
    C. Third generation cephalosporins are the most effective against gram-negative bacilli and B-lactamase.
    D. All cephalosporins are effective against anaerobic bacilli.

CRITICAL THINKING ACTIVITY

Why is there an increase in drug-resistant diseases?

What problems are produced by this trend?

Chapter 56
URINARY TRACT ANTISEPTICS

Definition of Terms

Define the following:

1. antiseptic

2. cystitis

3. glomerulonephritis

4. methenamine

5. nitrofurantoin

6. pyelonephritis

7. quinolone

8. urethritis

COMPLETION EXERCISE

QUINOLONES, NITROFURAN COMPOUNDS, AND METHENAMINES

Complete the table. The hints in parentheses are words within the terms used to fill the blanks. The hint words may have the letters in different order than they appear in the term. The terms will be much longer than the hints.

Quinolones	Nitrofuran Compound	Methenamines
Prototype: *Nalidixic Acid*	Prototype: *Nitrofurantoin*	Methenamine Hippurate
(ram) _____	10. (ant) _____, Furalan, Macrodantin	11. (hip) _____, Urex, Methenamine Mandelate
Pharmacotherapeutics		
2. Prevention and treatment of uncomplicated (sit) _____. Works against many urinary tract pathogens.	Treatment of UTIs caused by susceptible organisms.	Treat acute UTIs or suppress recurrent ones. 13. (log) _____ (met) _____ treatment of UTIs.
Pharmacodynamics		
14. Nalidixic acid binds to (and) _____and inhibits (and) _____ supercoiling and ultimately kills the bacterial cell wall.	Interferes with bacterial enzyme systems by inhibiting acetylcoenzyme A, which disrupts bacterial 15. (hot) _____ metabolism.	16. Forms (leer) _____ as it is hydrolyzed in the bladder. (leer) _____ has bacteriostatic action by denaturing bacterial proteins.
Contraindications and Precautions		
17. Severe (veil) _____ and kidney damage Convulsive disorders Children under 3 months	Oliguria 18. (sting) _____ (rot) _____ Pregnant clients near term Infants less than 4 weeks old 19. Debilitated or (bad) _____ clients	20. (head) _____ Renal insufficiency 21. (tap) _____ disease Asthma (Hiprex) Elderly, debilitated clients
Drug-Drug Interaction		
Oral 22. (long) _____	23. (lid) _____ acid 24. (data) _____ Uricosuric drugs 25. Drugs that delay (sag) _____ emptying	26. (USA) _____ microbials 27. Drugs that (kill) _____ the urine (sodium bicarbonate and acetazolamide)

UNDESIRED CLINICAL RESPONSES

For each undesired clinical response, identify the antibiotic (s) involved.

N=Nalidixic acids   F=Furodantin (nitrofurans)   M=Methenamines

28. _____   GI upsets

29. _____   Photosensitivity

30. _____   CNS headaches, dizziness, and visual disturbances

31. _____   Bladder discomfort

32. _____   Itchy rash

33. _____   Blood dyscrasias

34. _____   Progressive peripheral polyneuropathy

35. _____   Liver damage, hepatitis

36. _____   Brown or rusty colored urine

37. _____   Pulmonary hypersensitivity reactions

Complete the rationale for the following nursing interventions.

Nursing Intervention	Rationale
Clients on nalidixic acid and anticoagulants should have their prothrombin time monitored frequently.	38.
Clients on nalidixic acid or nitrofurantoin who are diabetic should be instructed to use a colorimetric test (Clinitest reagent strips or Tes-Tape) based on an enzyme reaction to test their urine for glucose.	39.
Clients on nalidixic acid should be advised to avoid direct sunlight or ultraviolet light while on the drug and for 3 months after it is discontinued.	40.
Clients on nalidixic acid or nitrofurantoin should be advised to avoid machinery and driving for a couple of days when beginning therapy.	41.
Infants under 1 month of age should not be given nitrofurantoin.	42.
Clients taking nitrofurantoin should be instructed to rinse the mouth well after swallowing the drug.	43.
Clients on methenamine should be taught to avoid alkaline food and consume an acid-ash diet.	44.
Clients on methenamine should be instructed to limit fluid intake of 1500 to 2000 mL per day.	45.

CRITICAL THINKING ACTIVITY

Mr. James Catado is an 82-year-old resident of the Valley View Long Term Care Center. His medical diagnoses include: frequent urinary tract infections, severe degenerative arthritis, NIDDM, and mild generalized arteriosclerosis. His arthritis is managed with acetominophen and NSAIDs. He also takes an oral antidiabetic drug and is on a 1,800 calorie ADA diet.

About 6 weeks ago, Mr. Catado was hospitalized for a TURP to treat benign prostatic hypertrophy. The frequent UTIs that Mr. Catado had prior to surgery have not resolved. Several attempts have been made to discontinue his catheter, but each time he becomes very distended and uncomfortable.

Identify the risk factors that are triggers for Mr. Catado's frequent infections.

The charge nurse receives an order for methenamine mandelate, 1 gram orally qid from Mr. Catado's physician. What about this order should be discussed further with the physician?

Do any potential drug-drug interactions exist in this situation?

CHAPTER 57
ANTIMYCOBACTERIAL DRUGS

ANTITUBERCULAR PROTOTYPE

Complete the following for INH (isonicotinic acid hydrazide).

Pharmacokinetics

1. After oral or IM administration, INH has _____ absorption.

2. Peak serum levels are achieved within ____ to ____ hours. If administered orally with food, tim

   to peak level is _____.

3. Metabolism of INH is _____ controlled. Asians and Eskimos metaboliz

   the drug _____ in comparison to Jews and Arabs.

Pharmacodynamics

4. INH is _____; the drug exerts its effect by interfering wit

   _____

FIRST-LINE ANTITUBERCULAR DRUG—RIFAMPIN

Complete the following for rifampin (Rimactane, Rifadin).

Pharmacodynamics

5. Rifampin is most active against _____ _____organisms.

   is both _____ and _____. Th

   drug inhibits _____ _____.

STUDY QUESTIONS

6. Explain what is meant by first-line and second-line antitubercular drugs. List three drugs fron
   each group.

7. For each antitubercular drug listed, provide common undesired responses and appropriate nursing measures, i.e., GI distress—administer the drug with food.

   a.   INH

   b.   rifampin

   c.   ethambutol hydrochloride

   d.   aminosalicylic acid

   e.   pyrazinamide

8. Provide the rationale for the following interventions.
Instruct the client receiving INH to avoid tyramine-containing and histamine-containing foods.
Rationale:

Monitor the results of liver function tests on clients receiving rifampin.
Rationale:

9. Why should the client receiving rifampin be advised against wearing soft contact lenses during therapy?

10. Why should the nurse assess the mucous membranes of a client receiving dapsone?

Multiple Choice

Select the best answer.

11. The nurse instructs the client receiving rifampin about common undesired clinical responses. These responses include:
  A. discoloration of body fluids.
  B. hair loss.
  C. discoloration of mucous membranes.
  D. hypertension.

12. The client receiving ethambutol should be assessed for:
  A. auditory changes.
  B. changes in visual acuity.
  C. flu-like symptoms.
  D. defects in blood clotting.

13. The client is receiving isoniazid. Which of the following vitamins would the client receive to prevent the peripheral neuritis that may accompany isoniazid therapy?
    A.   vitamin C
    B.   vitamin E
    C.   vitamin B_{12}
    D.   vitamin B_6

14. What is the mechanism of action for rifampin? The drug:
    A.   inhibits cell-wall biosynthesis.
    B.   interferes with synthesis of RNA.
    C.   impairs cell multiplication.
    D.   inhibits enzymes responsible for folic acid biosynthesis.

CRITICAL THINKING ACTIVITY

One of your clients, a 30-year-old Caucasian male, is being treated with isoniazid and rifampin for an *Mycobacterium tuberculosis* infection. His roommate, a 26-year-old African-American, has been prescribed isoniazid prophylactically.

Which of these individuals is likely to require vitamin B_6 supplementation? Why?

What specific instructions should be provided regarding the scheduling of rifampin doses?

Chapter 58
ANTIFUNGAL DRUGS

Definition of Terms

Define the following:

1. aspergillosis

2. azoles

3. blastomycosis

4. candidiasis

5. coccidioidomycosis

6. cryptococcal meningitis

7. cryptococcosis

8. dermatophyte

9. fluorinate pyrimidines

10. polygenes

11. rigors

12. superficial mycosis

13. systemic mycosis

14. tinea barbae

15. tinea capitis

16.   tinea corporis

17.   tinea cruris

18.   tinea pedis

19.   tinea unguium

20.   tinea versicolor

COMPLETION EXERCISE

21.   Candidiasis occurring in the oral cavity is called _____.

22.   Azole fungal agents may be divided into two categories, the _____ an
      the _____.

23.   The gold standard of therapy for treatment of systemic fungal infections is _____
      _____.

24.   An antifungal drug which is frequently administered with amphotericin B for the treatment
      cryptococcosis is _____.

25.   In clients receiving flucytosine, the serum concentration should be kept below _____ _____
      to avoid toxicity.

26.   Two drugs that should not be administered with drugs that decrease gastric acidity (such a
      antacids, H_2 blockers, or omeprazole) include _____ an
      _____.

27.   The nurse should instruct the client to take _____ with fatty foods t
      increase absorption of the drug.

28.   Clients with vulvovaginitis who are using antifungal agents should be told that to safely avoid in
      fecting their partners they should refrain from _____ _____
      until the course of therapy has ended.

STUDY QUESTIONS

29.   Which client populations are at particular risk for developing fungal infections?

30.   Which areas of the body are sites where candidiasis may occur?

1. What are appropriate nursing interventions for a client who has developed rigors following administration of amphotericin B?

2. What are appropriate nursing interventions for a client who is receiving fluconazole?

3. What are some common over-the-counter preparations for vulvovaginal candidiasis?

CRITICAL THINKING ACTIVITY

A client is receiving amphotericin B and flucytosine for a *Cryptococcus neoformans* infection. After 2 days of drug therapy, the client complains of nausea and diarrhea.

Why is this significant for this client?

What assessment measures should be addressed?

CHAPTER 59
ANTIVIRAL DRUGS

DEFINITION OF TERMS

Define the following:

1. infection phase

2. integration phase

3. interferons

4. nucleoside analogs

5. virion

Match the drug in column A with the usual indication from column B. Terms in Column B may be used more than once.

Column A		Column B	
6. ____ zidovudine		A.	Cytomegalovirus (CMV)
7. ____ acyclovir		B.	Human immunodeficiency virus
8. ____ ribavarin		C.	herpes simplex virus and herpes zoster virus
9. ____ amantadine		D.	hepatitis B and C
10. ____ zalcitabine		E.	herpes simplex keratitis
11. ____ interferon		F.	influenza
12. ____ didanosine		G.	respiratory syncytial virus
13. ____ idoxuridine			
14. ____ trifluridine			
15. ____ ganciclovir			
16. ____ vidarabine			

Indicate whether the following statements are true or false. Correct the false statements.

17. Acyclovir has been found to be an effective therapeutic adjunct in the treatment of chickenpox. True or False

18. Acyclovir may cause renal damage due to renal tubular precipitation and crystallization. True or False

19. An elevated platelet count is a potential adverse effect of acyclovir. True or False

20. Acyclovir cannot be given to the elderly client. True or False

21. Amantadine is only recommended after the onset of influenza symptoms. True or False

22. When ganciclovir is contraindicated in the treatment of CMV, foscarnet is the drug of choice. True or False

23. Clients receiving foscarnet are at high risk for renal dysfunction as well as fluid and electrolyte disturbances. True or False

24. A change in liver function tests would indicate intolerance to ganciclovir. True or False

25. OSHA mandates the disposal of unused portions of Acyclovir. True or False

26. Unused ophthalmic solutions of idoxiuridine should be kept in the refrigerator. True or False

27. Interferons have antineoplastic as well as antiviral properties. True or False

28. Clients receiving interferons may experience flu-like symptoms. True or False

29. The biggest controversy surrounding the administration of ribavarin is occupational exposure to health care providers and others. True or False

30. Ribavarin may be delivered safely to clients via a ventilator. True or False

31. Ribavarin has been reported to damage the contact lenses of health care workers exposed to it. True or False

32. Serious adverse effects have limited the use of vidarabine to the treatment of herpes simplex keratitis. True or False

STUDY QUESTIONS

33. Identify the primary mechanism of action of antiviral drugs.

34. What laboratory values need to be assessed when administering acyclovir?

35. List precautions to be initiated when giving acyclovir to an elderly client.

36. Differentiate between the therapeutic and prophylactic uses of amantadine.

37. Discuss the relevance of the nursing research conducted on amantadine.

38. Describe precautions to be taken when administering ganciclovir relative to OSHA guidelines.

39. Discuss how the dosing schedule for idoxiuridine may lead to noncompliance in clients. What are the implications for nursing.

40. Describe nursing measures that minimize the flu-like symptoms associated with the administration of the interferons.

CRITICAL THINKING ACTIVITY

Explain why vidarabine has been limited to the treatment of herpes simplex keratitis.

Chapter 60
ANTIPARASITIC DRUGS

Definition of Terms

Define the following:

1. cestode

2. helminths

3. nematode

4. parasites

5. protozoans

6. trematode

Match the mode of transmission with the parasitic agent. You may use the modes o transmission more than once.

7. ___	Hookworm	A.	Oral ingestion of poorly cooked fish, beef or pork
8. ___	Roundworm	B.	Person to person, fomites
9. ___	Malaria	C.	Flies
10. ___	Scabies	D.	Dogs, rabbits, cats, rats
11. ___	Liver fluke	E.	Contaminated water, raw vegetables
12. ___	Amebic dysentery	F.	Venereal
13. ___	Pneumocystis carinii	G.	Ingestion of raw or undercooked meat poultry, or dairy foods, oral contamina tion with cat feces
14. ___	Fish, beef, or pork		
15. ___	Trichomoniasis	H.	Person to person tapeworm
16. ___	Pediculus capitis—head lice	I.	Oral-fecal, self contamination
17. ___	Toxoplasmosis	J.	Fecal contamination of water or person t person
18. ___	Pinworm		
19. ___	Chiggers	K.	Oral ingestion of infected meat (pork)
20. ___	Maggots	L.	Female *anopheles* mosquito
21. ___	Lung fluke	M.	Skin penetration or inoculation
22. ___	Trichinosis	N.	Wooded, grassy areas, dogs, cats
23. ___	Blood fluke	O.	Inhalation
24. ___	Giardia diarrhea	P.	Oral ingestion of poorly cooked freshwate crab, crayfish, or raw fish
25. ___	Ticks		
26. ___	Pediculus pubis—pubic lice		

DRUGS USED TO TREAT HELMINTH INFECTIONS

List the main undesired clinical responses to anthelmintic drugs on the following body systems.

27. GI: _____

_____

28. CNS: _____

_____

29. Other: _____

_____

MULTIPLE CHOICE

Select the best answer.

30. The major groups of organisms that cause parasitic infections are:
    A. protozoa, nematodes, platyhelminthes, and arthropoda.
    B. bacteria, viruses, fungi, and spirochetes.
    C. cestodes, nematodes, prototodes, and platytodes.
    D. hookworms, roundworms, flatworms, and flukes.

31. Which statement is most accurate about the action of antiparasitic drugs?
    A. Mebendazole blocks glucose uptake by ectoparasites, depleting stores of glycogen and interfering with ability to reproduce.
    B. Thiabendazole suppresses egg or larval production in protozoa.
    C. Niclosamide inhibits energy production in the ova of cestode mitochondria.
    D. Praziquantel produces an increase in cell membrane permeability in susceptible trematodes.

32. Which antihelmintic drug should be avoided for clients with hepatic disease?
    A. mebendazole
    B. pyrantel
    C. dicarbamazine
    D. niclosamide

33. What antiparasitic drug may compete with other drugs for sites of metabolism in the liver and should be used with caution when given with other drugs because of the possibility of toxicity?
    A. thiabendazole
    B. niclosamide
    C. praziquantel
    D. metronidazole

34. Which sentence best describes antiparasitic drugs?
    A. Antiparasitic drugs are only given orally.
    B. Antihelminthic drugs tend to be more toxic than antiprotozoan drugs.
    C. Antiparasitic drugs often have GI upsets as undesired clinical responses.
    D. Antiparasitic drugs are organism-specific and do not treat different varieties of organisms.

35. Which answer is correct about antimalarial drugs?
    A. All of these drugs both prevent and treat the clinical disease.
    B. These drugs are safe enough to use during pregnancy and lactation.
    C. These drugs are only administered through IV infusions.
    D. Chloroquine phosphate is the main weapon against human malaria.

36. Which choice is most accurate about undesired clinical responses to antimalarial drugs?
    A. Mefloquine is the only antimalarial drug without GI side effects.
    B. At therapeutic doses, quinine produces a group of side effects known as cinchonism.
    C. Retinopathy may occur with long term quinine therapy.
    D. Tinnitus is an unusual clinical response to these drugs, indicating CNS involvement.

37. Which statement best describes contraindications and precautions to antimalarial drugs?
    A. Chloroquine and mefloquine are contraindicated in individuals with glucose-6-phosphate dehydrogenase deficiency.
    B. Primaquine is contraindicated in clients with impaired renal or hepatic function.
    C. Children and infants are extremely susceptible to adverse effects from parenteral chloroquine.
    D. Quinine should not be used concurrently with ß-blockers and calcium channel blockers.

CRITICAL THINKING ACTIVITY

Why are the non-drug teaching interventions just as important as the drug teaching interventions in people with parasitic infections?

Chapter 61

OVERVIEW OF FEMALE AND MALE REPRODUCTIVE SYSTEMS

Definition of Terms

Match the term in Column A with the correct definition in Column B.

Column A		Column B	
1. _____	estrogen	A.	male sex hormone
2. _____	cervix	B.	expulsion of seminal fluid from penis
3. _____	ovum	C.	female sex hormone
4. _____	orgasm	D.	release of ovum from ovary
5. _____	menarche	E.	cessation of menstruation
6. _____	testosterone	F.	production of mature sperm
7. _____	spermatogenesis	G.	lower part of uterus
8. _____	ejaculation	H.	female sex cell
9. _____	ovulation	I.	onset of menses
10. _____	menopause	J.	climax of the sexual response

Completion Exercise

11. The fertilized egg implants in the endometrium about _____ days after ovulation.

12. The process whereby sperm acquire the ability to fertilize ova is called _____.

13. The two stages of the male sexual response are _____ _____ _____ and _____.

STUDY QUESTIONS

14. At what age do the reproductive organs of the male become functionally mature? Of the female?

15. Which hormones do the following:
    a. stimulates ovarian follicle to start forming:

    b. sharp rise causes follicle to ovulate:

    c. stimulates proliferation of the endometrium following menstruation:

    d. stimulates growth of ducts of mammary glands:

    e. decreases motility of uterus:

16. Describe the hormonal changes that occur during the normal menstrual cycle.

17. Trace the development of a mature sperm from its beginnings as a spermatogonium to ejaculation.

MULTIPLE CHOICE

Select all correct answers.

18. Testes produce which of the following?
    A. ICSH
    B. testosterone
    C. sperm
    D. LH
    E. FSH

19. Testosterone secretion is controlled by:
    A. FSH.
    B. LH.
    C. ICSH.
    D. TSH.
    E. ACTH.

20. A ruptured ovarian follicle becomes:
    A. a corpus luteum.
    B. an ectopic pregnancy.
    C. a corpus spongiosum.
    D. a site of progesterone production.

21. Fertilization most often occurs:
    A. 12 to 15 days after ovulation.
    B. in the fallopian tube.
    C. the day after intercourse.
    D. in the vagina.
    E. at the cervix.

Chapter 62
DRUGS AFFECTING THE FEMALE REPRODUCTIVE SYSTEM

Definition of Terms

Define the following:

1. anovulation

2. basal body temperature

3. biphasic

4. hypoestrogenic

5. monophasic

6. progestin

7. triphasic

HYPOTHALAMIC STIMULANT PROTOTYPE

Complete the following information about gonadorelin acetate (Lutrepulse).

8. Gonadorelin acetate is indicated in the treatment of _____ produced by a defect in the secretion of _____ from the hypothalamus.

9. Gonadorelin acetate stimulates the release of _____ and _____ in the anterior pituitary gland.

10. Gonadorelin acetate is administered by _____ IV doses to mimic the

_____.

The recommended course of treatment is 21 days.

OVULATORY STIMULANT PROTOTYPE

Complete the following information about clomiphene citrate (Clomid).

11. Clomiphene citrate is indicated for the induction of _____.

12. Clomiphene citrate has both _____ and _____
     properties. The drug binds to estrogen receptors, causing the _____
     _____ to respond as if there is an estrogen deficit. This response stimulates the release
     of ____ and____ , resulting in ovulation.

HYPOTHALAMIC INHIBITOR PROTOTYPE

Complete the following information about leuprolide acetate (Lupron Depot)

13. Leuprolide acetate is indicated for the treatment of _____ and
     _____ _____.

14. This drug constantly _____ the anterior pituitary gland to secrete____
     and _____. With prolonged administration, pituitary receptors become _____
     and subsequent ____ and ____ secretion is suppressed. As a result, estrogen production is
     _____.

STUDY QUESTIONS

15. Provide the rationale for the following nursing interventions.
     Teach the client receiving estrogen therapy to avoid excessive sunlight.
     Rationale:

     Clients receiving therapy with oral anticoagulants must be monitored carefully if estrogen therapy
     is started.
     Rationale:

     Instruct the client receiving estrogen therapy that breast and pelvic examinations are recom-
     mended every 6 to 12 months.
     Rationale:

16. What is the primary pharmacotherapeutic use for oral synthetic progestins? Describe the
     pharmacodynamic properties of progesterone. What are major undesired clinical responses
     associated with exogenous progesterone therapy?

7. What is unique about the progestin, levonorgestrel? Develop a teaching plan for a client scheduled to receive levonorgestrel therapy.

8. Differentiate among monophasic, biphasic, and triphasic oral contraceptive pills.

MULTIPLE CHOICE

Select the best answer.

9. Oxytocin is prescribed for your client. The pharmacotherapeutic uses for this drug include:
   A. induction of labor.
   B. relaxation of the myometrium.
   C. inhibition of prostaglandin synthase.
   D. inhibition of uterine contractions.

20. Inhibition of uterine motility and of labor may be caused by administration of:
   A. vasopressin.
   B. methylergonovine maleate.
   C. dinoprostone.
   D. ritodrine hydrochloride.

21. When is uterine muscle responsiveness to oxytocin most prominent?
   A. during the first trimester of pregnancy
   B. during the second trimester of pregnancy
   C. near or at term
   D. during all stages of pregnancy

22. Which one of the following is a prominent side effect associated with the therapeutic use of estrogens?
   A. osteoporosis
   B. sodium retention
   C. confusion
   D. parkinsonism

CRITICAL THINKING ACTIVITY

A friend is expecting her first baby in a few months. She does not want to breast feed and asks you about the use of drugs to inhibit lactation. She asks specifically about chlorotrianisene (Tace).

What should be your response to your friend? What should you tell her about the drug chlorotrianisene? What measures could you suggest to decrease postpartum breast engorgement?

CHAPTER 63
DRUGS AFFECTING THE MALE REPRODUCTIVE SYSTEM

DEFINITION OF TERMS

Define the following:

1. anabolic steoids

2. anabolism

3. androgens

4. catabolism

5. testosterone

6. List four therapeutic uses for androgens:

_____

_____

_____

_____

Match the drug with the appropriate characteristic. You will only have one answer for each characteristic.

T=Testosterone   M=Methyltestosterone   N=Nandrolone   D=Danazol

7. _____   Used to treat endometriosis

8. _____   Results in an increased risk of atherosclerosis

9. _____   Has increased anabolic and decreased androgenic properties

10. _____   Produces cholestatic hepatitis and jaundice

11. _____   Interferes with glucose tolerance and iodine uptake diagnostic tests

12. _____   The standard drug of comparison for the other three.

For each system describe undesired clinical responses common to therapy with androgens.

13. Integumentary system:

14. Hematologic system:

15. GI system:

16. Urinary system:

17. Skeletal system:

18. Reproductive system, males:

19. Reproductive system, females:

20. Other:

Provide the rationale for the following nursing interventions.

Nursing Intervention	Rationale
Monitor cholesterol levels of clients on methyltestosterone.	21.
Monitor weight of clients on androgens.	22.
Monitor prothrombin levels of clients on androgens and anticoagulants.	23.
Monitor diabetic clients on androgens closely for alterations in blood glucose levels.	24.
Monitor women on danazol who have migraines or epilepsy for fluid retention.	25.

Indicate if the statement is true or false. Correct the false statements.

26. ____   Concurrent administration of androgens with ACTH and corticosteroids enhances the tendency for nausea.

27. ____   Androgen therapy is contraindicated for women and children, of either sex, except for specific indications.

28. ____   All androgens are classified as Pregnancy Category X drugs.

29. ____   Androgens should be given with caution in individuals with a history of drug abuse

30. ____   There are three subcategories of androgens: androgens, anabolic steroids, and catabolic steroids.

31. ____   Antiandrogen drugs are used to treat prostatic neoplasms since these tumors are androgen dependent.

32. ____   Serum prostate specific antigen levels are effective screening tools for prostatic cancer for those clients taking finasteride.

33. ____   Severe side effects of long-term anabolic steroid use are impaired liver and renal function.

CRITICAL THINKING ACTIVITY

You are requested to present a program on abuse of anabolic steroids for a high school physical education class. What specific information about the problems of abusing anabolic steroids do you think would most impress the students? Why?

CHAPTER 64
DRUGS USED IN OCULAR DISORDERS

DEFINITION OF TERMS

Define the following:

1. allergic conjunctivitis

2. blepharitis

3. chalazion

4. cycloplegia

5. fungal keratitis

6. glaucoma

7. hordeolum

8. intraocular pressure

9. keratitis

10. miosis

11. mydriasis

STUDY QUESTIONS

12. Describe the procedure for instilling eye drops.

13. Describe the procedure for instilling eye ointment singularly and in combination with eye drop

14. Differentiate between eye solutions and eye suspensions. Describe actions that should be take prior to instillation of either a solution or a suspension.

Match the statement in Column A with the appropriate term in Column B.

Column A   **Column B**

15. ____ main medication action is pupil-   A.   Cyclogyl
          lary dilatation
                                                B.   cromolyn sodium
16. ____ causes a greenish discoloration
          around any torn conjunctival epi-   C.   Ophthalgan
          thelium
                                                D.   mydriatic
17. ____ commonly used beta-adrenergic
          blocking agent   E.   sympathomimetic mydriatics

18. ____ medication that paralyzes muscles   F.   fluorescein
          of accommodation
                                                G.   Timoptic
19. ____ ophthalmic hyperosmotic drug
                                                H.   Stoxil
20. ____ antiviral ophthalmic drug
                                                I.   Hypotears
21. ____ ophthalmic drug used to treat ocu-
          lar allergic responses   J.   fluorescein angiography

22. ____ used for aqueous deficiency

23. ____ skin may have yellowish tone for 6
          to 12 hours after use

24. ____ contraindicated in clients with nar-
          row angle glaucoma

CRITICAL THINKING ACTIVITY

Mydriacyl 0.5% solution, 1 gtt O.U., is to be administered 10 minutes prior to an ophthalmic examination. If you were the nurse, what actions would you perform?

What instructions would you give the client regarding the effects of the drug and precautions to follow after the examination?

The elderly client, who is to instill an eye medication b.i.d., lives alone and has osteoarthritis and tremors. Describe alternative techniques that can be taught to the client for self-administration of eye medication.

Chapter 65
EAR PREPARATIONS

Definition of Terms

Define the following:

1. cerumen

2. furuncles

3. ototoxicity

4. pinna

5. tragus

Study Questions

6. Summarize elements to be assessed during examination of the ear.

7. Describe the procedure for irrigating an ear.

8. Describe the procedure for administering ear drops. What age-related factor must be considered when instilling ear drops into the external ear canal?

9. Provide the rationale for the following nursing interventions.
   Warm otic preparations before administration.
   Rationale:

   Manipulate the pinna up and backward when instilling ear drops in adults.
   Rationale:

   Local anesthetics should not be used in children <1 year of age.
   Rationale:

10. List five drugs that can lead to ototoxicity.

Match the statement in Column A with the appropriate drug in Column B. Each statement in Column A has only one correct answer.

Column A		Column B	
11. _____	Used for the treatment of external otitis	A.	benzocaine
12. _____	Used for relief of inflammation of external canal	B.	acetic acid-Burrow's solution
13. _____	Used to emulsify cerumen	C.	desonide-acetic acid
14. _____	Used to alleviate pain	D.	chloramphenicol otic
15. _____	Used as antibacterial, drying agent	E.	carbamide peroxide

Match the ear disorder to its anatomic site.

16. _____	tympanic perforation	A.	external ear
17. _____	Meniere's disease	B.	middle ear
18. _____	furuncles	C.	inner ear
19. _____	otitis media		
20. _____	cerumen		

MULTIPLE CHOICE

Select the best answer.

21. An 8-year-old client with a severe external ear canal infection is prescribed chloramphenicol 0.5% otic solution. What is the usual dosage for this condition?
    A.   1 drop into ear canal daily
    B.   2 drops bid into ear canal
    C.   2 to 3 drops tid or qid into ear canal
    D.   3 drops every 3 hours into ear canal

22. During a routine physical assessment, the client complains of decreased hearing in his/her right ear. Inspection of the ear canal reveals impacted cerumen. Which one of the following conditions would contraindicate the use of carbamide peroxide?
    A.   Meniere's disease
    B.   perforated tympanic membrane
    C.   labyrinthitis
    D.   otitis media

23. A solution that can be used to irrigate th ears is:
    A.   full strength hydrogen peroxide.
    B.   full strength ethyl alcohol.
    C.   50% ethyl alcohol.
    D.   Burrow's solution.

CRITICAL THINKING ACTIVITY

A client is scheduled to receive an ototoxic drug. What actions must the nurse take before initiating drug therapy?

Two to 3 days after drug therapy has started the client complains of hearing disturbance. What nursing actions are appropriate?

CHAPTER 66
LOCAL ANESTHESIA

DEFINITION OF TERMS

Define the following:

1. caudal block

2. epidural block

3. eutectic mixture

4. intravenous regional block

5. local anesthesia

6. local infiltration

7. peripheral nerve block

8. saddle block

9. spinal block

10. surface coolant

11. topical anesthetic

STUDY QUESTIONS

12. What factors determine the rate of absorption of a local anesthetic?

13. Why is epinephrine used as an additive to local anesthesia?

   When is epinephrine contraindicated?

14. Why is a test dose of a local anesthetic administered after an epidural catheter is inserted?

   What are signs of incorrect catheter placement?

15. Name several clinical uses for each of the following routes of administration.
   a. surface (topical) anesthesia

   b. infiltration anesthesia

   c. epidural (caudal) anesthesia

16. What are some common hypersensitivity reactions associated with local anesthesia?

MULTIPLE CHOICE

Select all correct answers.

17. A client receiving an epidural anesthetic should be monitored for which of the following:
   A. hypotension
   B. respiratory depression
   C. leakage from catheter side
   D. urinary retention

18. Local anesthetics commonly used for local infiltration include:
   A. lidocaine
   B. bupivacaine
   C. procaine
   D. cetacaine

19. Undesired clinical responses associated with local anesthetics include:
   A. restlessness
   B. tachycardia
   C. headache
   D. nausea

CRITICAL THINKING ACTIVITY

Mrs. Wagner comes to the office to have some skin lesions removed from her back and right arm. The primary care provider plans to do shave biopsies of the lesions using lidocaine hydrochloride with epinephrine as the local anesthetic. The procedure should last approximately 20 minutes.

What information would be important to obtain from Mrs. Wagner during the preanesthetic history?

In preparing the local anesthetic for injection, why should the vial and solution be examined?

Mrs. Wagner expresses some anxiety about the anesthesia. She asks the nurse if the anesthetic will paralyze her arm or make her sleepy. How should the nurse respond?

At the conclusion of the procedure, what information should the nurse give Mrs. Wagner that is specific to the local anesthetic?

CHAPTER 67
DRUGS USED TO TREAT DERMATOLOGIC CONDITIONS

DEFINITION OF TERMS

Define the following:

1. acne vulgaris

2. dermis

3. epidermis

4. keratinocyte

5. melanocyte

6. psoriasis

7. scabies

8. vitiligo

ACNE PREPARATIONS

Match the characteristic with the correct acne preparation. Each drug has more than one answer; use the characteristics more than once.

	Drugs		Characteristics
9. _____	isotretinoin (Accutane)	A.	Oral administration only
10. _____	tretinoin (Retin-A)	B.	Topical use only
11. _____	benzoyl peroxide	C.	Both oral and topical use
12. _____	tetracycline	D.	Suppresses inflammation and growth of *P. acnes*
13. _____	erythromycin		
14. _____	clindamycin (Cleosin)	E.	Reduces population of *P. acnes*, inhibits chemotaxis, and decreases the percentage of free fatty acids in the skin

F. Decreases sebum production and composition, inhibits *P. acnes* growth, inhibits inflammation, and alters patterns of keratinization

G. Reduces the amount of keratin in sebaceous follicles and inhibits chemotaxis, phagocytosis, complement activation, and cell-mediated immunity of bacteria

H. Increases the rate of sloughing of epithelial cells and destroys comedomes

I. Increases cell turnover of epidermis and decreases cohesiveness of keratinized cells decreasing formation of existing comedomes and inhibiting formation of new ones

Describe nursing interventions directed at helping clients manage undesired clinical responses of acne preparations.

15. Photosensitivity from isotretinoin (Accutane) or tretinoin:

16. Dryness and irritation of skin from tretinoin or benzoyl peroxide:

17. GI upset with oral clindamycin or erythromycin:

18. Teratogenic fetal CNS defects with isotretinoin:

DRUGS USED TO TREAT PSORIASIS

Match the action with the appropriate drug or therapy.

19. ____ etretinate (Tegison)

20. ____ methotrexate sodium

21. ____ coal tar

22. ____ anthralin

23. ____ calcipotriene

24. ____ topical corticosteroids

25. ____ phototherapy

26. ____ methoxsalen

A. Inhibits DNA synthesis by binding with DN
Decreases epidermal proliferation by inhibiti
mitochondrial activity

B. Upon photoactivation, probably conjugates a
forms covalent bonds with DNA

C. Inhibits synthesis in rapidly proliferating e
dermal cells. Works on the S phase, the pha
of a large number of psoriatic cells

D. Appears to inhibit keratinization, proliferatio
and differentiation of epithelial cells and
inflammatory

E. Modifies the functions of epidermal and derm
cells and of leukocytes participating in prol
erative and inflammatory skin diseases

F. Used with UVA light therapy and acts to cau
transient corticosteroids epidermal hyperplas
that lasts 1-2 weeks, followed by cytostasis a
epidermal thinning. Light activates to preve
further epidermal cell replication and increa
prostaglandin synthesis in the skin.

G. Inhibits DNA synthesis and stimulates mel
nin pigmentation.

H. Inhibits proliferation and enhances differenti
tion of human keratinocytes

Match the drug with correct administration information.

27. ____ calcipotriene

28. ____ topical corticosteroids

29. ____ etretinate (Tegison)

30. ____ phototherapy

31. ____ anthralin

32. ____ methoxsalen

33. ____ methotrexate sodium

34. ____ coal tar

A. Orally with fatty food or milk to increase a
sorption

B. Orally 1 hour before or 2 hours after meals
parenterally

C. Topically with thin coating; avoid contact wi
the face

D. Use disposable gloves when applying topicall
apply sparingly and wash off with soap a
water after 15-20 minutes therapy

E. Must be combined with a photosensitizing age
to be beneficial

F. Topically apply after shower or bath for be
absorption; do not apply to weepy denude
areas

G. Topically may be used with anthralin cream

H. Orally with food or milk or topically

MULTIPLE CHOICE

Select the best answer.

5. Which statement is most accurate about characteristics of the skin?
   A. Stratum corneum cells are important because they manufacture histamine.
   B. Mast cells are important because they contain the anticoagulant heparin.
   C. In Caucasians, melanin is distributed throughout the epidermis.
   D. The dermal layer is important for temperature regulation.

36. Which answer best describes undesired clinical responses to antifungal drugs?
   A. Ketoconazole may cause conjunctivitis and chelitis.
   B. Undecylenic acid causes GI upset.
   C. Photosensitivity may result from undecylenic acid.
   D. Cross-sensitivity to penicillin exists with griseofulvin.

CRITICAL THINKING ACTIVITY

What are the ethical considerations with the use of isotretinoin as an acne treatment for young women?

CHAPTER 68
OVERVIEW OF NORMAL AND NEOPLASTIC CELL GROWTH

DEFINITION OF TERMS

Define the following:

1. anaplastic

2. carcinogenesis

3. cell cycle

4. differentiation

5. DNA

6. doubling time

7. generation time

8. interphase

9. latency period

10. mitosis

11. oncogenes

12. proto-oncogenes

13. RNA

14. undifferentiated

15. well-differentiated

STUDY QUESTIONS

16. What is the role of DNA in cell growth?

17. Name the main phases of the cell cycle. Briefly describe the main activity during each of these phases.

18. Some cells don't go through the cycle but stop in a resting phase. What factors contribute to this occurrence?

19. Describe three ways in which benign tumor cells differ from malignant tumor cells.

20. Give four environmental factors that can act as carcinogens.

21. The primary care provider must consider several factors when selecting an antineoplastic agent. Describe some of the factors that should be considered.

MULTIPLE CHOICE

Select the best answer.

22. Which one of the following is the genetic matter of the cell?
    A.   DNA
    B.   RNA
    C.   protein
    D.   ribosomes

23. The site of cellular protein synthesis is the:
    A.   lysosome.
    B.   mitochondria.
    C.   ribosome.
    D.   endoplasmic reticulum.

24. Cells reproduce themselves through a process called:
    A.   meiosis.
    B.   mitosis.
    C.   protein synthesis.
    D.   replication.

25. The main cell part that regulates movement of substances into and out of the cell is the:
    A.   cytoplasm.
    B.   nucleus.
    C.   cell membrane.
    D.   endoplasmic reticulum.
    E.   centriole.

CHAPTER 69
ANTINEOPLASTIC DRUGS

DEFINITION OF TERMS

Define the following:

1. alopecia

2. benign

3. cycle specific drug

4. cytotoxic

5. drug resistance

6. malignant

7. metastasis

8. mitotic inhibitor

9. mucositis

10. myelosuppression

Match the following drug groups with the appropriate description of their action.

11. _____ Alkylating agents

12. _____ Alkaloids

13. _____ Antibiotics

14. _____ Antimetabolites

A. replaces correct building materials, i.e., purine, amino acids, with antagonists

B. replaces H ion in a substance with alkyl group

C. blocks transcription of new DNA or RNA

D. blocks cell division in metaphase

The most common undesired clinical responses to chemotherapeutic drugs are nausea and vomiting, mucositis, alopecia, and bone marrow suppression. **For each of these responses identify appropriate nursing interventions.**

Nausea and Vomiting	Mucositis	Alopecia	Bone Marrow Suppression

For each of the following routes of administration, list at least three nursing interventions.

Intrathecal	Intravenous Piggyback	Intravenous Bolus	Oral

For each of the following antineoplastic drug categories, list the prototype.

Category	Prototype
Alkylating Agent	
Antimetabolites	
Antibiotics	
Hormones	

STUDY QUESTIONS

5.   Name four factors that limit the effects of chemotherapy.

6.   Why is it important for a client to have a healthy immune system when receiving chemotherapy treatment?

7.   Why are multiple courses of chemotherapy necessary?

8.   When a cancer client is receiving chemotherapy, what are the general effects that you would expect to observe?

CRITICAL THINKING ACTIVITY

You are caring for a client on Actinomycin D. He develops stomatitis. What nursing actions should you take?

You are the nurse in an oncology clinic. A new client is to begin therapy on Leukeran. What should be your initial actions?

Chapter 70
FLUID, ELECTROLYTE AND NUTRITIONAL BALANCE

Definition of Terms

Locate the answers to the following clues in the word puzzle on the following page.

1. Amount of heat needed to raise the temperature of 1 gram of water 1 degree Celsius.

2. Nutrient providing the chief source of energy in most diets.

3. Vitamins A, D, E, and K (3 words).

4. Form of carbohydrates that circulates in the bloodstream; only source of energy for the central nervous system.

5. Excess carbohydrates are converted to this substance; substance stored in liver or converted into fat.

6. Calories expressed for nutritional requirements.

7. Nutrient that provides a concentrated source of energy ; spares protein as an energy source.

8. Foods that contain the elements necessary for body function.

9. Organic compounds necessary to regulate metabolic processes; act as catalysts.

10. Level of intake of essential nutrients considered adequate to meet the needs of healthy individuals.

11. Vitamins C and B complex (2 words).

12. Nutrient necessary for life that is present in all body tissues.

13. Calcium, chloride, magnesium, potassium, sodium, and phosphorus. Daily amounts >100 mg required.

14. Chromium, cobalt, copper, fluorine, iodine, iron, zinc, manganese, molybdenum, and selenium.

O E E I M F D Z A J Q Q L O R I P F S

J S W B P N M A C R O M I N E R A L S

G L Z D W V D C E Z F Y S Y Z T A K E

B Z P E U R I S Y D Q A K B - R G W I

H A G L Y C O G E N G D T S E Y Y R R

F G N B N C F Z R D Q H O N V M R S O

C O T U U N K D B X V L I P I D M E L

E L C L T S F P D C U M I S K T E Y A

G T G O X R C A B O H Y D R A T E C

I S I S K L I L L R X Q O E S J D Y O

M Q U - I L F E C V N S T J H E Z N L

C A F R V C V I N G D W R T F M C X I

Y T P E Z I M V H T R Y E T B M T O K

K A N T T T N R V Q S J S U U D D C O

J W G A E K P V W I S P C F U V W E P

E L M W W W N V C D A U I M V O E G E

J I N G Z Z I M J B B P C Q K O O Z N

N D C B B V I Z V F S M S A D N A Y Q

Y K K R R O B A I T U O A W W T F I A

W Q I A L B T A G L R V D O S W I M V

CHAPTER 71
FAT-SOLUBLE VITAMINS

FAT-SOLUBLE VITAMIN DEFICIENCY

Match the signs and symptoms of vitamin deficiency with the appropriate vitamin. You wil **have from 4 to 6 answers per vitamin. You will use each answer only once.**

1. _____ Vitamin A

2. _____ Vitamin D

3. _____ Vitamin E

4. _____ Vitamin K

A. reproductive failure

B. hemorrhage

C. decreased corticosteroid production

D. muscular dystrophy, myopathies

E. hypocalcemia or hypophosphatemia

F. GI bleeding, epistaxis, hematuria

G. night blindness, corneal and conjunctiva dryness, corneal ulceration

H. secondary hyperparathyroidism

I. follicular hyperkeratosis

J. retinal degeneration

K. proximal muscle weakness

L. prolonged bleeding and clotting times

M. hemolytic anemia

N. growth failure, faulty bone and tooth development

O. bone pain or tenderness

P. fetal malformations

Q. bruise easily

R. moderate to severe neurologic abnormal ties

S. impaired resistance to infections.

T. poor bone demineralization; rickets in chi dren and osteomalacia in adults

Match the risk factors with the vitamin deficiency. You may use answers more than once.

5. _____   Vitamin A

6. _____   Vitamin D

7. _____   Vitamin K

8. _____   Vitamin E

A.   B-Thalassemia major

B.   individuals with diseases that alter fat digestion and absorption such as sprue, cystic fibrosis, bowel resections, chronic diarrhea, inflammatory bowel disease, short bowel syndrome

C.   hemorrhagic disease of newborn

D.   high intake of polyunsaturated fatty acids

E.   prematurity

F.   selenium deficiency

G.   chronic renal disease

H.   impaired liver storage or cirrhosis

I.   hypoparathyroidism, hyperthyroidism

J.   alcoholism

K.   children under age of 5 years with poor diet

L.   biliary or pancreatic problems

FAT-SOLUBLE VITAMIN TOXICITY

Determine which type of toxicity the symptoms represent: acute vitamin A, chronic vitamin A, acute vitamin D, or chronic vitamin D

9._____

Urinary: Polydipsia, polyuria

Hematologic: Leukopenia

Skeletal: Cortical thickening on bones, deep bone pain, arthralgias, premature epiphyseal closure, slow skeletal growth

CNS: Headache, irritability progressing to psychiatric symptoms, pseudotumor cerebri

Integumentary: Changes texture of hair, nails, cheilitis, and cheilosis desquamation, dry, cracking skin, gingivitis, hyperpigmentation, pruritus alopecia

Gastrointestinal: Anorexia, weight loss, hepatosplenomegaly, jaundice, ascites

10. _____

Cardiovascular: Cardiac arrhythmias, hypercholesterolemia

CNS: Overt psychosis, hyperthermia

Kidney: Renal failure

Integumentary: Pruritus, soft tissue calcification

Gastrointestinal: Pancreatitis

Reproductive: Decreased libido

Visual: Photophobia, rhinorrhea,

11. _____

Renal: Nephrocalcinosis, proteinuria, polydipsia and polyuria
CNS: Headache, mental status changes
Cardiovascular: Hypertension
Gastrointestinal: Constipation, dysgeusia (bad taste), anorexia, diarrhea, vomiting
Circulatory: Hypercalcemia

12. _____

CNS: Drowsiness, irritability, headache, vertigo, blurred vision, bulging fontanel in children
Gastrointestinal: Abdominal pain, anorexia, nausea, vomiting
Circulatory: Hypercalcemia in adults

Identify the common causes of toxicity for each vitamin.

13. Vitamin A:

14. Vitamin D:

15. Vitamin E:

16. Vitamin K:

NURSING CONSIDERATIONS

Indicate if the statement is true or false. Correct the false statements.

17. ____   Vitamin D is absolutely contraindicated in pregnancy because of its teratogenic effect
resulting in deformities of head, face, and genitourinary system.

18. ____   Vitamin D increases serum calcium levels, so clients on digoxin and vitamin D shoul
be monitored closely for signs of digoxin toxicity.

19. ____   Nurses should monitor prothrombin times closely for clients on vitamin A.

20. ____   Newborn infants delivered to hypercalcemic mothers should be monitored closely fo
hypocalcemia.

21. ____   Concurrent use of vitamin D with magnesium antacids in chronic renal dialysi
clients may lead to hyperkalemia.

22. ____   Clients with liver failure should be monitored carefully for signs of of osteomalaci
because of decreased ability to hydroxylate cholecalciferol to active form.

23. ____   Anaphylactic and allergic reactions may occur with IV dosing of vitamin A. Hypersen
sitive reactions such as urticaria may occur at injection sites.

MULTIPLE CHOICE

Select the best answer.

24. Which is the best example of pharmaco-therapeutics for fat-soluble vitamins?
    A. Vitamin A is used for prevention or control of bronchopulmonary hyper-plasia and retrolental fibroplasia in premature infants who require high concentrations of oxygen.
    B. Vitamin D diminishes the risk of toxic effects from vitamin A.
    C. Vitamin K_1 is considered the safest K supplement for premature or low birth weight neonates.
    D. Large doses over short periods of time are most effective for Vitamin A deficiency.

25. Which statement is most accurate about toxicity of fat-soluble vitamins?
    A. Coumarin, clofibrate, and salicylates can cause vitamin K toxicity.
    B. The greatest risk for vitamin E toxicity is when taken in combination with selenium.
    C. Vitamin D toxicity may be confused with hypercalcemia from other causes.
    D. Vitamin E has a toxic effect on infants when given in IV infusion.

26. Which answer is correct about vitamin K_3?
    A. It is considered relatively safe to use with neonates and premature infants.
    B. It is a natural form of vitamin K.
    C. It is used for hypoprothrombinemia caused by hepatic failure or genetics.
    D. It is not safe to use during pregnancy.

27. Which choice best describes the physiology of vitamin K and E?
    A. Vitamin K is distributed through body tissues with tissue concentrations directly proportional to fat content of tissue.
    B. Both vitamin K and E require the presence of bile salts for absorption.
    C. K_3 is produced by intestinal flora and released into gut lumen.
    D. Vitamin E is rapidly mobilized from adipose and muscle stores in deficiency states.

CRITICAL THINKING ACTIVITY

What is the rationale for adding vitamins A, D, and E to the IV solution as close to infusion time as possible?

Chapter 72
WATER-SOLUBLE VITAMINS

Definition of Terms

Define the following:

1. angular stomatitis

2. beriberi

3. bioflavonoids

4. carnitine

5. cheilosis

6. choline

7. glossitis

8. inositol

9. paraaminobenzoic acid

10. pellagra

11. pernicious anemia

12. pyridoxine-dependent infant

13. scurvy

14. tobacco amblyopia

IGNS OF DEFICIENCY FOR WATER-SOLUBLE VITAMINS

Match the cluster of deficiency symptoms with the appropriate vitamin. Use each answer only once.

5. _____ Ascorbic acid

6. _____ Thiamin (*dry beriberi*)

7. _____ Thiamin (*wet beriberi*)

8. _____ Thiamin (*Wernicke's*)

9. _____ Riboflavin

0. _____ Niacin

1. _____ Pantothenic acid

2. _____ Pyridoxine

3. _____ Cobalamin

4. _____ Folic acid

5. _____ Biotin

A. Dermatitis, diarrhea, and dementia

B. Pernicious anemia, GI lesions, constipation, bilateral paresthesia of fingers and feet, and spastic ataxia

C. Anorexia, nausea, vomiting, glossitis, mental depression, alopecia, and dermatitis

D. Decreased muscular strength and onset of peripheral and central neuropathies

E. Megaloblastic, macrocytic anemias, malabsorption syndromes, spina bifida and anencephaly in the neonate

F. "Burning feet" syndrome—numbness, tingling and burning of feet and hands

G. Physical fatigue, weakness, loss of appetite, petechial (spot) hemorrhages, follicular hyperkeratosis, swelling and bleeding gums, bleeding around hair roots

H. Loss of memory, disorientation, and confabulation

I. High-output heart failure and edema

J. Angular stomatitis or cheilosis, sore throat, hyperemic oral mucosa, glossitis, anemia, seborrheic dermatitis, itching or burning of eyes, and visual problems

K. Irritability, depression, nervousness, seizures, peripheral neuropathies, seborrheic skin rash, and anemia

URSING CONSIDERATIONS

Describe the rationale for the following nursing actions.

6. Monitor clients with megaloblastic anemia who have a poor dietary intake or a history of CHF carefully for the first week of replacement therapy with cobalamin.

27. Monitor clients carefully who are on phenytoin therapy for seizures if folate supplementation is begun.

28. Emphasize the importance of regularly receiving monthly cobalamin injections to clients who have previously had deficiencies and are still at risk for deficiencies.

29. Clients on prolonged folic acid supplementation should be monitored closely for signs of cobalamin deficiency.

30. Clients with zinc deficiency should be monitored for folic acid deficiency.

31. Pyridoxine should not be given with levodopa.

Develop nursing interventions for each of the following situations.

32. Ascorbic acid and folic acid are sensitive to heat.

33. Riboflavin increases the rate of degradation of folic acid in IV solutions, especially when exposed to ultraviolet light. Thiamin and biotin are also sensitive to light.

34. Vitamin C may cause stomach upset.

35. Vitamin C may interfere with the absorption of copper.

36. A client on nicotinic acid is complaining of flushing of the face, neck, and chest.

MULTIPLE CHOICE

Select the best answer.

37. Which symptoms would be most indicative of pyridoxine toxicity?
    A. dry mouth, increased sebaceous gland activity and burning, stinging or tingling skin
    B. nausea, vomiting, heartburn, hunger pains, bloating, flatulence, and diarrhea
    C. ataxia, decreased vibratory sense, and decreased proprioception
    D. dizziness, syncope, blurred vision, transient headache, nervousness, and panic

38. Which statement is most accurate about toxicity of water-soluble vitamins?
    A. Toxic reactions are most likely to occur with synthetic cobalamines.
    B. There are no reports of toxicity for thiamin.
    C. Toxic reactions are rare but serious for biotin.
    D. Toxic reactions are common for ascorbic acid and pantothenic acid.

39. Which answer best describes water-soluble vitamin deficiencies?
    A. Cobalamin deficiency anemias and neurologic damage resolve slowly if at all.
    B. Those at highest risk for biotin deficiency are young women on oral contraceptives.
    C. Water-soluble deficiencies are rare because these vitamins are stored in fat.
    D. Fatal thiamin deficiency can develop in as short of time as three weeks.

40. Which sentence is correct?
    A. Nicotinamide has no direct vitamin activity.
    B. Nicotinic acid is the active form of niacin.
    C. Nicotinamide is used to treat pellagra.
    D. Nicotinic acid is used to treat persons with nicotine dependency.

CRITICAL THINKING ACTIVITY

During the assessment interview on admission, a pregnant woman indicates that she has been taking high doses of pyridoxine during pregnancy. What additional data do you need to collect?

Does this situation present any potential problems for the fetus?

The newborn?

CHAPTER 73
MINERALS

DEFINITION OF TERMS

Define the following:

1. apotransferrin

2. cretinism

3. fluoritosis

4. fluorosis

5. glucose tolerance factor

6. goiter

7. heme

8. hemochromatosis

9. macromineral

10. micromineral

11. pica

12. transferrin

13. Wilson's disease

For each of the following minerals, indicate if it is a macromineral (A) or micromineral (B) by placing the appropriate letter in the space before each mineral.

14. ____ calcium

15. ____ chromium

16. ____ chloride

17. ____ cobalt

18. ____ copper

19. ____ fluorine

20. ____ magnesium

21. ____ iodine

22. ____ iron

23. ____ potassium

24. ____ sodium

25. ____ manganese

26. ____ phosphorus

27. ____ molybdenum

28. ____ selenium

29. ____ zinc

IRON

30. Signs and symptoms of iron deficiency anemia include: _____

_____.

31. _____ _____ is the most common oral iron preparation.

32. Indications of iron toxicity include:_____.

33. _____ _____ is used to treat iron poisoning.

ZINC

34. Indications of zinc deficiency include: _____

_____.

35. Sources of dietary zinc include: _____.

IODIDE

36. Iodide deficiency is associated with the formation of a _____.

37. Additional indications of iodide deficiency include: _____

_____.

38. Sources of dietary iodine include: _____.

For each of the minerals listed, provide the mechanism of action and indications of deficiency.

Mineral	Mechanism of Action	Indications of Deficiency
Chromium		
Copper		
Selenium		
Manganese		
Fluorine		
Molybdenum		
Zinc		

CRITICAL THINKING ACTIVITY

A female client informs you that she plans to discontinue birth control measures so that she can try to conceive. What specific prenatal minerals are considered essential?

Chapter 74

Agents Affecting the Volume and Ion Content of Body Fluids

Definition of Terms

Match the fluid imbalance in the first column with its description in the second column.

Fluid Imbalance		Description
1. ____ fluid volume excess	A.	Fluid is retained in excess of electrolytes, or solutes are lost more rapidly than fluids
2. ____ fluid volume deficit		
3. ____ hypo-osmolar imbalance	B.	Fluid and solutes are gained in isotonic proportions
4. ____ hyperosmolar imbalance	C.	Fluid is lost in excess of solutes, or solutes are gained more rapidly than fluids
	D.	Fluid and solutes are lost in isotonic proportions.

Completion Exercise

Complete the following table by listing two causes and one treatment for each of the fluid imbalances.

Fluid Imbalance	Causes	Treatment
Fluid Volume Excess		
Fluid Volume Deficit		
Hyperosmolar Imbalance		
Hypo-osmolar Imbalance		

List the changes in laboratory data expected when a client experiences each of the osmola **fluid imbalances.**

Imbalance	Serum Sodium	Serum Osmolality	Hematocrit	Blood Urea Nitrogen
Hyperosmolar Imbalance				
Hypo-osmolar Imbalance				

5. List the normal serum level for each of the following electrolytes:

   a.   sodium

   b.   potassium

   c.   magnesium

   d.   calcium

   e.   phosphorus

6. Provide the use(s) for the following dextrose in water solutions:

   a.   D5W/D10W

   b.   D25W

   c.   D50W

Find the words that match the statement. The words may appear diagonally, horizontally, vertically, or backwards.

```
A  Y  T  I  L  A  L  O  M  S  O  G  H  J  M
I  I  W  D  I  O  L  L  O  C  R  A  Y  X  Y
S  O  M  E  Y  Z  O  M  L  A  A  L  P  D  A
O  N  E  E  L  S  P  W  N  D  S  B  E  I  I
T  C  L  F  S  G  H  U  E  E  I  U  R  O  M
O  O  W  S  X  E  L  M  L  L  S  M  T  L  E
N  T  O  T  O  O  N  Z  P  Q  O  I  O  L  R
I  I  G  V  C  P  U  G  U  D  M  N  N  A  T
C  C  N  Y  N  K  S  M  A  K  S  Y  I  T  A
T  T  T  Q  J  P  R  H  A  M  O  X  C  S  N
Z  E  P  N  A  R  T  X  E  D  R  O  V  Y  O
S  H  Y  P  O  T  O  N  I  C  E  E  Q  R  P
H  Y  P  O  K  A  L  E  M  I  A  S  P  C  Y
B  I  C  A  R  B  O  N  A  T  E  L  T  Y  H
H  Y  P  E  R  O  S  M  O  L  A  R  Q  N  H
```

7. A protein product given to expand vascular volume or reduce edema.

8. Combines with hydrogen ions to treat metabolic acidosis.

9. Intravenous solution that contains protein or starch molecules.

10. An intravenous solution that does not contain protein or starch molecules.

11. A plasma expander.

12. A blood component used to treat neutropenia.

13. Exists when the serum magnesium is greater than 2.5 mEq/L.

14. A fluid imbalance in which the fluid in the vascular space is more concentrated than the fluid in the intestinal and intracellular spaces.

15. The tonicity of a fluid space that draws water into it.

16. Exists when the serum potassium is less than 3.5 mEq/L.

17. Sodium imbalance that can result from the gain of water into the extracellular compartment or the loss of solutes.

18. When this tonicity exists in a fluid space, the space will contract or shrink as fluid moves out.

19. Occurs when the concentrations of fluids on two sides of a semi-permeable membrane are equal.

20. The vascular pressure, primarily determined by serum albumin, that holds fluid in the vascular space.

21. The concentration of intravascular fluids.

22. The movement of water across a semi-permeable membrane in response to differences in concentration.

Match the blood product in the first column with its therapeutic use in the second colum
Each therapeutic use can be used more than once.

Blood Product	**Therapeutic Use**
23. ____ Red blood cells	A. reduce risk for infection
24. ____ Fresh frozen plasma	B. replace vascular volume; improve oxyge carrying capacity of blood
25. ____ Factor VIII	
26. ____ Platelets	C. prevent or treat bleeding
27. ____ Granulocytes	
28. ____ Immune globulin	

Match the transfusion reaction in the first column with the cause in the second colum

Transfusion Reaction	**Cause**
29. ____ hemolytic reaction	A. sensitivity to donor's white cells, platelet or plasma proteins
30. ____ anaphylactic reaction	
31. ____ febrile, nonhemolytic reaction	B. ABO-incompatible blood was administere
32. ____ allergic reaction	C. infusion of IgA proteins to individual wi IgA antibodies
	D. sensitivity to donor's plasma protein

CRITICAL THINKING ACTIVITY

Indicate the significance of the following observations in a client receiving intravenous fluids.

Shortness of breath:

Moist rales:

Bounding pulse:

Hypertension:

CHAPTER 75
ENTERAL AND PARENTERAL NUTRITIONAL THERAPY

DEFINITION OF TERMS

Find the words that match the statement. The words may appear diagonally, horizontally, vertically, or backwards.

```
D  M  D  E  Z  I  R  E  D  N  E  L  B  L  L
H  S  O  P  O  L  Y  M  E  R  I  C  I  A  A
P  C  E  D  M  P  T  Y  M  H  B  P  R  N  K
R  G  A  T  U  V  V  R  N  U  I  E  T  I  N
O  L  W  M  A  L  H  T  P  D  T  H  Y  S  O
C  U  Z  H  O  R  A  I  S  N  R  R  B  O  I
A  C  E  D  L  T  D  R  E  O  N  V  O  T  T
L  E  L  T  J  U  S  Y  P  N  L  P  L  O  A
A  R  D  B  Z  L  P  O  H  E  U  B  X  N  R
M  N  R  O  V  R  M  A  X  O  J  L  F  I  I
I  A  E  P  O  E  W  F  D  F  B  H  I  C  P
N  W  R  T  T  Y  X  G  H  X  J  R  U  G  S
E  M  E  R  E  N  E  T  I  R  E  M  A  V  A
B  I  I  U  M  S  I  L  O  B  A  N  A  C  X
N  C  S  L  A  R  E  N  I  M  O  R  C  A  M
```

1. Process in which body tissues are replaced and repaired and new tissue growth takes place.
2. Non-invasive methods to indirectly measure nutrition.
3. Complication of tube feedings in which formula enters the respiratory tract.
4. Tube feeding formula made by transformation of intact food to a liquid consistency.
5. This nutrient must be broken down to monosaccharides in order to be absorbed by the gastrointestinal tract.
6. The administration of nutrients into the gastrointestinal tract.
7. An example of a tube feeding formula designed for use by clients with diabetes mellitus.
8. The nutrient that provides the most concentrated source of energy.
9. Electrolytes that are required in daily amounts greater than 100 mg.
10. An example of a milk-based polymeric tube feeding formula.
11. A single nutrient product that may be given alone or in combination with other nutrients.
12. Tube feeding solutions that contain all the essential nutrients in complex form.
13. An example of a product that can be given as peripheral parenteral nutrition.
14. Food sources of this nutrient include dairy products, meat, and eggs.

Study Questions

15. List one advantage and two disadvantages of small-bore pliable feeding tubes.

16. Explain the rationale for using a large vein for administration of parenteral nutrition.

17. Describe nursing interventions that can be used to prevent bacterial contamination of tube feeding equipment or formula.

18. List five topics that need to be included in the teaching plan of a client scheduled to receive enteral or parenteral nutrition in the home.

Multiple Choice

Select the best answer.

19. In parenteral nutrition formulas, calories are provided by a combination of carbohydrate and lipid administration in order to:
    A. prevent hypoglycemia.
    B. foster catabolism.
    C. minimize growth of muscle mass.
    D. spare protein for use in anabolic processes.

20. TPN solutions are initiated slowly in order to:
    A. allow adaptation to the increase in glucose and osmolality.
    B. prevent infection.
    C. prevent fluid volume deficit.
    D. reverse the negative nitrogen balance.

Describe the procedure, advantages, and disadvantages of each type of tube feeding listed below.

Type of Schedule	Procedure	Advantages	Disadvantages
Bolus			
Intermittent			
Continuous			

CRITICAL THINKING ACTIVITY

When hypertonic liquid medications are administered to a client receiving a tube feeding, what nursing intervention should be performed to prevent diarrhea?

CHAPTER 76
ANTISEPTICS, DISINFECTANTS, AND STERILANTS

DEFINITION OF TERMS

Define the following:

1. antiseptic

2. asepsis

3. bactericide

4. bacteriostatic

5. clean technique

6. disinfectant

7. germicide

8. medical asepsis

9. sterilant

10. sterile technique

11. sterilization

12. surgical asepsis

Match the agent listed in Column A with the category in Column B. Agents may have more than one answer and categories in Column B are used more than once.

	Column A		Column B
13. _____	hexachlorophene	A.	antiseptic
14. _____	cresol	B.	disinfectant
15. _____	gentian violet	C.	bactericidal
16. _____	silver nitrate	D.	bacteriostatic
17. _____	hydrogen peroxide	E.	sterilant
18. _____	ethanol		
19. _____	formaldehyde		
20. _____	ethylene oxide		

Identify which of the following measures are components of sterile technique (S) or clean technique (C)

21. _____ hand washing

22. _____ steam autoclave

23. _____ pasteurizing milk

24. _____ washing surface of table with soap and water

25. _____ gowning and gloving for surgical procedure

26. _____ gowning and gloving for client with decreased leukocytes

27. _____ inserting Foley catheter for urine specimen

CRITICAL THINKING ACTIVITY

One evening while you are caring for clients in the emergency department, a a 20-year-old male is admitted with nausea and vomiting. During your assessment, you note several skin lesions on the man's arms and legs.

According to Universal Precautions what actions must you take while caring for this individual? Why?

Chapter 77
DRUGS USED TO MANAGE POISONING

Definition of Terms

Define the following:

1. emetics

2. gastric lavage

3. ipecac

Study Questions

4. What drugs are most often responsible for poisoning of children?

5. Identify major components of accidental poisoning prevention.

6. What should you teach clients regarding the management of poisoning victims at home? What action must be taken initially?

7. List the components of care of the poisoned client at the hospital.

8. What is the action of ipecac syrup? Of activated charcoal? In what situations are these drugs administered?

CRITICAL THINKING ACTIVITY

You are on duty when the mother of a 3 year old calls the emergency department. She fears that her child has swallowed some "old medicine" that was stored in the medicine cabinet.

What are the initial questions that you ask the mother?

How might you determine if emergency room treatment is necessary?

Following the emergency situation, what would you teach the mother about accidental poisoning?

CHAPTER 78
DRUGS USED FOR DIAGNOSTIC PROCEDURES

DEFINITION OF TERMS

Define the following:

1. barium sulfate

2. intradermal test

3. isotope

4. opacity

5. patch test

6. provocative

7. radioisotope

8. radiopaque agent

9. scratch test

10. tuberculin anergy

Complete the following table by providing information on desired action, clinical use, and interpretation.

Agent	Clinical Use	Desired Action	Interpretation
Tuberculin			
Histoplasmin			
Mumps skin test allergen			

STUDY QUESTIONS

1. What are some nursing considerations regarding the following imaging agents?
   a. barium sulfate

   b. diatrizoate meglumine (ionic iodinated compound)

   c. metrizamide (nonionized iodinated compound)

   d. iocetamic acid (oral cholecystographic compound)

2. List five major provocative agents and their clinical use.

3. Describe the mode of action of in vivo markers and tracers. What are major therapeutic uses for these diagnostic agents?

CRITICAL THINKING ACTIVITY

Develop a teaching plan for the following nursing diagnoses: Anxiety related to lack of knowledge regarding histoplasmin skin test and Bowel elimination, alteration in: constipation related to barium ingestion.

Answer Keys

CHAPTER 1

11. natural
12. laxatives, purgatives
13. Pharmacology
14. documents
15. Hippocrates
16. drugs
17. textbooks
18. remedies
19. minerals
20. pharmacopeia
21. herbs
22. toxicity
23. Paracelsus
24. native
25. science
26. site
27. action
28. plant
29. microbial
30. environmental
31. D
32. C

CHAPTER 2

1. to 5. Check textbook for definitions.
6. D
7. E
8. B
9. C
10. A
11. 5
12. 3
13. 3
14. 1
15. 2
16. 4
17. 1
18. 2

19. C
20. D
21. B
22. A
23. C
24. A
25. B

CHAPTER 3

1. Resins
2. Excipients
3. Glycosides
4. Disintegration
5. Gums
6. Oils
7. Dissolution
8. Alkaloids
9. Active ingredients
10. Pharmaceutic phase
11. C
12. E
13. A
14. F
15. B
16. D
17. B
18. D
19. A
20. B

CHAPTER 4

20. D
21. C
22. B
23. A
24. False—Only free, unbound drug molecules cross the cell membrane.
25. True
26. True

27. False—Low serum concentrations of free-unbound drug decreases absorption.
28. True
29. False—The microsomal enzyme system of the liver is responsible for metabolizing most drugs.
30. True
35. C
36. B

CHAPTER 5

12. True
13. False—Drugs that produce their effects by interacting with enzymes are considered structurally specific drugs.
14. True
15. True
16. False—Drug potency refers to the relative amount of a drug required to produce the desired response.
17. False—The relationship between the drug dose administered and the response generated is the dose-response curve.
23. B
24. C

CHAPTER 6

1. F
2. N
3. I
4. K
5. G
6. D
7. A
8. J
9. M
10. B
11. L
12. O
13. E
14. H
15. C
25. A
26. C
27. B
28. A
29. B
30. D
39. Ototoxicity
40. Carcinogenesis

CHAPTER 7

4. modified
5. distribution, biotransformation
6. acidic, alkaline
7. combined action of drugs at receptor sites.
8–14. Examples are available within the text book.
19. C
20. B

CHAPTER 8

6. True
7. False— A 20-gauge needle is used for intramuscular injections.
8. False—A vial usually contains more than one drug dose.
9. False—Air does not need to be added to an ampule before withdrawing the drug.
10. False—Oil used as a vehicle slow downs the absorption of drugs.
11. True
12. J
13. F
14. E
15. C
16. D
17. K
18. B
19. G
20. H
21. I
22. L
27. C
28. B
29. D
30. D
31. C
32. A

CHAPTER 9

1. D
2. F
3. A
4. E
5. C
6. G

7. B
8. Biologic
9. health, illness
0. Family
1. Time
2. control
3. C
4. D
5. B
6. A
7. D
8. C
9. A
20. B
21. D
22. C

CHAPTER 10

1. observable
2. stimuli
3. verbal
4. perceptions
5. negatively
6. beliefs
7. response
8. illness
9. B
10. D
11. A
12. D
13. C
14. A
15. C

CHAPTER 11

1. Herbalism
2. Acupressure
3. Self-medication
4. Homeopathy
5. Self-administration
6. Acupuncture
7. Self-treatment
8. B
9. A
10. C

CHAPTER 12

1. D
2. H
3. B
4. F
5. E
6. G
7. J
8. A
9. L
10. I
11. C
12. K
18. Stomach
19. Small intestine
20. Food, milk
21. 2, 6
22. Liver
23. Protein
24. Norepinephrine
25. Inhibitory
26. Excitatory
27. Central nervous system
28. Acetaldehyde
29. Antabuse
30. Acetaldehyde
31. Powder
32. Snorting, inhalation
33. Short
34. Liver
35. 15, 30
36. Cortical
37. Catecholamine
38. Norepinephrine
39. Fibrillation
40. Respiratory
41. Hyperactive
42. Neurotransmitters
43. Withdrawal symptoms
44. Tetrahydrocannabinal
45. Flowering tops
46. Resin
47. Marijuana
48. Hash
49. THC

50. Liver
51. Lungs
52. Fatty tissues
53. Metabolites
54. Neurons
55. Respiratory
56. Reproductive

CHAPTER 13

1. teratogen
2. lactation
3. myoepithelial cells
4. embryonic period
5. colostrum
6. prolactin
7. organogenesis
8. fetal period
9. oxytocin
10. ovum
11. cell differentiation
15. caffeine, nicotine, and alcohol consumption during pregnancy
16. facial dysmorphology, prenatal and postnatal growth deficiencies, and central nervous system involvement
17. abruptio placentae, premature birth, growth retardation, low birth weight, neurobehavioral problems
18. plasma drug concentration, mammary metabolism, characteristics of drugs, stage of breast feeding, and amount of milk produced
21. Food and Drug Administration, American Academy of Pediatrics
22. C
23. A
24. D
25. C
26. C

CHAPTER 14

1. Puberty
2. Physical growth
3. 11
4. 19
5. First month
6. First year
7. Newborn
8. Birth
9. 28th day
10. 3
11. 6
12. 6
13. Puberty
19. Some drugs have better absorption with alkalinity. Acid-labile drugs may not be adequately absorbed.
20. Prolonged gastric emptying time, irregular and unpredictable peristalsis
21. Altered drug absorption
22. Low lipase concentrations and reduced concentration of bile acid
23. Enhanced percutaneous absorption
24. Increased permeability
25. Irregular absorption from subcutaneous and intramuscular sites
26. D
27. A
28. C
29. B

CHAPTER 15

Seek and Find Words:

```
N  B  X  P  Z  H  D  V  S  G  P  C
T  M  I  T  E  L  D  E  R  L  Y  S
A  G  Q  R  V  N  O  R  M  A  L  E
I  X  E  K  E  L  L  Y  N  P  P  N
P  D  T  R  A  V  J  E  O  I  A  E
O  C  M  F  I  X  Y  L  D  N  H  S
Y  T  H  O  M  A  S  D  J  N  K  C
B  R  E  W  J  Q  T  E  U  E  L  E
S  T  Y  U  A  I  O  R  A  L  S  N
E  K  J  H  C  G  F  L  I  L  D  C
R  L  M  N  O  B  V  Y  X  C  Z  E
P  R  E  S  B  Y  C  U  S  I  S  T
Y  C  A  M  R  A  H  P  Y  L  O  P
```

1. polypharmacy
2. elderly
3. very elderly
4. senescence
5. geriatrics
6. presbyopia
7. presbycusis

12. A
13. B
14. D
15. B

CHAPTER 16

1. Following a treatment regimen properly.
2. Working with other disciplines on behalf of clients towards common goals.
3. Failure to adhere to a therapeutic regimen because of an informed decision.
4. Decisions about the relative importance of various factors.
6. Complete on your own. Remember client outcomes are what tell you how effective your nursing interventions were!
7. The need for multiple venous punctures, rotation of intravenous site, pain, sclerosis of veins, and clotting at the site of insertion.
8. Potential for infection, catheter occlusion, thromboocclusion and extravasation

CHAPTER 17

1. Resting potential
2. Neuroglia
3. Neurotransmitter
4. Polarization

5. Action potential
6. Synapse
7. Threshold potential
8. Neuron
9. Depolarization
14. G
15. I
16. L
17. F
18. P
19. M
20. S
21. A
22. B
23. N
24. R
25. H
26. O
27. D
28. E
29. K

30. C
31. Q
32. J
33. B
34. A
35. D

CHAPTER 18

1. 60 minutes
2. 8 to 12 hours
3. 10 to 12 hours
4. liver
5. 53 to 118 hours
6. kidneys; 25 to 50 %
7. 80 to 90 %
8. highly
9. 15 to 45 minutes; 3 to 4 hours
10. 1 to 2 hours
11. 20 to 100 hours
12. B
13. C
14. A
16. Low dose of diazepam decreases total volume and respiratory rate; excessively high doses produces significant respiratory depression.
21. Onset of action is 15 to 45 minutes; effects diminish in 3 to 4 hours.
24. A
25. C
26. D
27. A
28. B

CHAPTER 19

1. O
2. R
3. E
4. K
5. S
6. T
7. J
8. N
9. Q
10. B
11. C
12. G

13. H
14. I
15. D
16. F
17. L
18. A
19. M
20. P
21. 10 to 30 minutes
22. 15 to 30 minutes
23. 4 to 5 hours
24. liver
25. kidneys, trace
26. mu, delta
27. 2 to 5 minutes
28. competitive, mu, kappa, sigma, delta
34. C
35. B
36. B
37. A

CHAPTER 20

11. erratically, unpredictably
12. lungs, liver, adrenal glands, spleen
13. slowly; 24
14. dopamine, acetycholine, histamine, norepinephrine
15. 8 to 23
16. 2 to 6; 72
17. 80 to 90%; 12 to 16
29. C
30. A
31. D
32. C
33. A

CHAPTER 21

1. C
2. D
3. F
4. B
5. A
6. E
7. small intestine
8. 90%

9. 1 1/2 to 12 hours; 22 hours
0. extensively
1. motor cortex; sodium
2. 10 to 20 µg/ml
3. 30; 60
4. 20 to 25%; 40 to 50%
5. 30 to 180 minutes; 10 to 20 days
6. 30 days
24. D
25. C
26. C

CHAPTER 22

6. brain; central nervous system
7. 4 to 24
8. enantiomers
9. oral route
18. D
19. C
20. D

CHAPTER 23

11. B
12. A
13. D
14. C
15. A
16. D
17. Levodopa (L-dopa, Dopar, Larodopa)
18. Carbidopa
19. Amantadine (Symmetrel)
20. Bromocriptine mesylate (Parodel), cabergoline, pergolide mesylate (Permax)
21. Benztropine mesylate (Cogentin)
22. Catecholamine
23. Levodopa
24. Tremors
25. On-off
26. Rapid
27. Tolerance
28 Dopamine
29. Cannot
30. Slows
31. GI tract
32. Dopamine
33. Unknown

34. Early
35. Orthostatic hypotension
36. Dyskinesia
37. Reversible
38. Legs, arms
39. Dysrhythmia
40. Psychotic
41. Liver
42. Epilepsy
43. Congestive heart failure
44. Hypertensive crisis
45. Levodopa
46. Antidepressants
47. Undesired
48. Glucose
49. Asians
50. Blood pressure
51. Orthostatic hypotension
52. Several hours before bedtime
53. Congestive heart failure
54. Drowsiness

CHAPTER 24

8. C
9. B
10. C
11. A
12. B
13. B
14. A
15. A

CHAPTER 25

18. parasympathetic and sympathetic nervous system
19. cholinergic
20. adrenergic
21. acetylcholine, norepinephrine, epinephrine
27. C
28. C

CHAPTER 26

11. decrease
12. decrease
13. decrease

14. relax
15. relax
16. relax
17. relax
18. dilate
19. decrease
20. no effect
21. decrease
30. increase secretions
31. increase mucus secretion; bronchospasm
32. contraction of iris
33. increase peristalsis and secretions
34. contract detrusor, relax trigone
35. decrease rate and force
36. dilate
37. dilate
49. B
50. C
51. A
52. C

CHAPTER 27

5. decrease
6. decrease
7. contract
8. constrict
9. contract
10. contract
11. relax
12. increase
13. increase
14. dilate
15. relax
16. increase
17. F
18. D
19. G
20. C
21. A
26. C
27. D
28. C
29. B
30. C
31. D

CHAPTER 28

5. See page 313 in text
6. 1 minute; 2 to 5 minutes; 35 to 60 minutes
7. acetylcholine; nicotinic binding
8. 30 seconds; 1 minute; 4 to 10 minutes
9. pseudocholinesterase
10. 5 hours
11. 3 hours
12. 8.7 hours; 7.3 hours

CHAPTER 29

11. Superior vena cava
12. Aorta
13. Right pulmonary artery
14. Left pulmonary artery
15. Right pulmonary vein
16. Left pulmonary vein
17. Right atrium
18. Left atrium
19. Pulmonic valve
20. Aortic valve
21. Mitral valve
22. Parietal pericardium
23. Pericardial space
24. Visceral pericardium
25. Epicardium
26. Myocardium
27. Endocardium
28. Inferior vena cava
29. Tricuspid valve
30. Right ventricle
31. Left ventricle
32. Descending aorta
33. D
34. C
35. A
36. E
37. B
46. B
47. C
48. A

CHAPTER 30

4. 30 to 60 minutes; 12 to 24 hours
5. 1 to 4 minutes
6. preload; afterload; systolic; resistance
7. readily
8. 1 to 2 hours
9. 90%
17. C
18. A
19. C
20. D

CHAPTER 31

8. passive; dosage form
9. slowed
10. 30 to 120 minutes; 2 to 6 hours
11. 1 1/2 to 2 days
20. C
21. A
22. B
23. C

CHAPTER 32

1. D
2. E
3. F
4. G
5. A
6. H
7. B
8. C
9. D
10. A
11. F
12. B
13. C
14. B
15. D
16. E
17. C
18. G
26. D
27. A
28. C
29. B

CHAPTER 33

6. Baseline blood pressure, pulse, and weight are measured. Then convert weight to kilograms
7. Yes. 50 mg/500 mL provides 100 mcg/mL of nitroprusside. The maximum dose is 10 mcg/kg/minute. At 68 kg, the maximum dose for Mr. Jamieson is 680 mcg/kg/minute or 6.8 mL/minute. The drug is infusing at 500 mcg/minute.
8. The nurse should ask the client what drugs he has used in the past to control blood pressure and address the specific drug that caused the problems, if possible. If this information is not known, the nurse should acknowledge that this effect may occur with some antihypertensives. The nurse should stress the need for continued therapy to prevent complications of hypertension. (See Chapter 30.)
9. African-Americans tend to have low plasma renin hypertension, so ACEI drugs that inhibit renin as the primary method of action are less effective in this population.
11. drowsiness, sedation
12. clonidine (Catapres)
13. Apply the transdermal system to a hairless area of intact skin on upper arm or torso, once every 7 days. Use a different site with each application and remove the old system. If the system loosens during the week, apply the adhesive overlay directly over the system. Check for skin irritation when the system is removed.
14. Rebound hypertension. Instruct clients to take the drug as prescribed and not to stop the drug or alter dosage except under supervision of the prescriber. Advise them of the rebound phenomenon which, with some agents, may not occur for 2 to 4 days after therapy is abruptly stopped.
16. orthostatic symptoms
19. elderly and African-Americans
20. CHF, asthma, IDDM, PVD, hypertriglyceridemia
21. Monitor BP and ECG continuously during infusion. Monitor BP at 5 minutes intervals for 30 minutes after infusion, then at 30 minute intervals for 30 minutes, then at 30 minute intervals for 2 hours and then hourly for 6 hours.
22. norepinephrine depletors
23. Depression, which may persist well after drug is discontinued, may occur.
38. B
39. A
40. C
41. D

CHAPTER 34

14. Heparin has an antithrombin effect. It binds to plasma cofactor and destroys thrombin and Factor X. It inhibits conversion of prothrombin to thrombin and has antithromboplastic effects.

17. Warfarin decreases concentration of prothrombin. It interferes with action of vitamin K; prevents synthesis of clotting factors.

22. H, W, HW, W, W, HW

23. Binding bile acids and inhibiting their reabsorption and enterohepatic cycling; LDL; constipation, heartburn, nausea, vomiting, vitamin deficiencies

24. water; Intense flushing

25. interfering with cholesterol synthesis; lovastatin, fluvastatin, simvastatin, pravastatin sodium

26. production of thromboxane A_2; platelet aggregation

27. streptokinase; dissolving intravascular fibrin clots; intracranial bleeding

28. B

29. C

30. A

31. D

CHAPTER 35

10. A, D

11. C, D

12. C, E, A, D

13. A, D

22. C

23. D

24. D

CHAPTER 36

10. E, F

11. F

12. D

13. C

14. G

15. H

16. A, H

17. B

18. A, F

19. A, D

20. B

21. rapidly; 2 hours; 4 hours; 6 to 12 hours; 5 to 14 hours; 61%

22. distal convoluted tubules; sodium and chloride; potassium and magnesium

23. decrease; uric acid

24. well; 95 %; 30 to 60 minutes; 1 to 2 hours; 4 to (hours

25. 5 minutes; 2 to 3 hours

26. rapidly; 1 to 3 hours; 30 to 180 minutes; 3 to 10 hours

27. nonabsorbable; osmolarity; water; sodium and chloride

28. Proximal convoluted tubule - osmotic diuretics and carbonic anhydrase; Ascending limb of the loop of Henle—loop diuretics; Distal convoluted tubule —thiazide diuretics; Terminal distal convoluted tubule - potassium-sparing diuretics; Cortical collecting duct —potassium sparing diuretics

32. B

33. B

34. C

35. C

CHAPTER 37

9. rapidly; 2 to 4 hours; 6 to 12 hours

10. urate; uric acid; double

11. well; 2 to 3 hours; oxypurinol; 18 to 20 hours

12. skin rash; diarrhea, nausea, increased serum alkaline phosphatase, increased aspartate aminotransferase and alanine aminotransferase

17. A

18. C

19. D

20. A

CHAPTER 38

1. D

2. A

3. F

4. C

5. E

6. B

7. H

8. G

9. D

10. B

11. C

12. I

13. F

14. A
15. E
16. False. Release of thyroid hormones is regulated primarily by negative feedback.
17. True.
18. False. Thyroid hormones increase the rate of activity in all body tissues, which increases the BMR. This increases metabolism.
19. False. Thyroid hormones increase the permeability of cell membranes to sodium and potassium
20. True.
21. False. Calcitonin is produced only when there is excess calcium is in the blood. It inhibits bond resorption of calcium and allows excretion in the urine.
22. False. Parathormone promotes the formation of the hormone calcitriol, an active form of vitamin D.
23. True.
24. Alpha
25. Beta
26. Raises
27. Lowers
28. More
29. Synthesis
30. Storage
31. Synthesize
32. Store
33. Accelerates
34. Gluconeogenesis
35. Stimulate
36. Transport
37. Transport
38. Increases

CHAPTER 39

15. False. Hypoglycemia can cause brain damage, not pancreatic damage.
16. False. Insulin-dependent diabetes mellitus (IDDM, type I) results from insufficient insulin production. IDDM requires daily insulin injections.
17. False. The opened vial that the client currently using should be stored at room temperature and used within 4 to 6 weeks. Cold insulin has a decreased absorption rate. Surplus insulin should be stored in the refrigerator.
18. False. Exercise does increase the use of serum glucose, but insulin dosage is not decreased. Exercise should occur at least 20 minutes after a meal and be at a consistent time and level.

19. True. Lipertrophy or lipohypertrophy occur at the sites of repeated insulin injections.
20. True.
21. False. It is not considered accurate because of differences in renal thresholds. Serum levels are considered accurate.
22. False. Sediment in the bottom is common with modified insulin preparations. The vial should be gently inverted several times or rotated to suspend the sediment into the solution.
23. False. Clients should not change their brands either. Any change in insulin may result in a need to adjust dosage.
24. A, E, I, L, M
25. C, D, F, G, J
26. B, D, G, H, K
27. B, G
28. E, G
29. F, H
30. C, H
31. A, H
32. D, H
33. Reactions; hypoglycemia
34. Parenterally
35. Rash; hypokalemia
36. Glucose
37. Diazoxide
38. Glucagon
39. D
40. D
41. A
42. C

CHAPTER 40

8. vasopressin
9. corticotropin
10. somatrem
11. somatrem
12. vasopressin
13. corticotropin
14. somatrem
15. corticotropin
16. vasopressin

CHAPTER 41

10. 50 to 80%
11. liver and kidneys

12. 6 to 7 days; 2 to 3 weeks
13. increasing; gluconeogenesis; growth, differentiation
14. rapidly
15. 30 minutes; 2 hours
16. inhibits synthesis of thyroid hormones
17. parenterally
18. 15 minutes; 4 hours; 24 hours
19. calcium; calcium; phosphorous; sodium

CHAPTER 42

1. C
2. F
3. D
4. A
5. G
6. B
7. E
8. Adrenal insufficiency; secondary adrenal
9. Immunosuppressive
10. inflammatory
11. Respiratory
12. Psychosis
13. Glaucoma
14. Peptic ulcer
15. Increased
16. Increased
17. Fats
18. Increased
19. Hyper
20. Decreased
21. Mobilization
22. Suppression
23. Adrenal
24. Sodium
26. Potassium
26. Retention
27. Calcium
28. Osteoporosis
29. Weakness
30. Muscle
31. Adrenal; Rheumatoid arthritis
32. Adrenocortical
33. GI tract
34. Prednisolone
35. Kidneys
36. Glucocorticoid
37. Proteins
38. Immune
39. Inflammatory
40. Glucocorticoid
41. Renal; chloride; potassium
42. A
43. C
44. B

CHAPTER 43

7. D
8. E
9. C
10. A
11. B
12. larynx
13. trachea
14. right
15. cigarette smoke
16. terminal
17. surfactant
18. active; passive
19. negative
20. accessory
21. resistance; increases
22. decreased
23. from; capillary
24. higher; alveoli
25. oxygen

CHAPTER 44

1. Rhinitis
2. Nasal congestion
3. Paradoxical reaction
4. Congested and nonproductive
5. Allergic rhinitis
6. Dry and nonproductive
7. Rebound phenomenon
8. Sinusitis
9. Cold
10. Congested and productive
11. Stomatitis
12. Mucous membranes
13. Middle ear infections
14. Histamine
15. Respiratory tract

6. Chronic diseases
7. Viscosity
8. Dry, nonproductive
9. Liquefies
10. Viscid
11. C
12. A
13. D
14. C

CHAPTER 45

6. Agonist
7. Receptors
8. Tachycardia
9. Vasodilator
10. Diaphragm; mucous
11. Coronary artery
12. Diabetes mellitus
13. Respiratory
14. Peptic ulcer
15. Paradoxical bronchospasm
16. Oppose
17. Additive
18. Increases
19. Contraceptives
25. A
26. A
27. B
28. A
29. B
30. B
31. A
32. B
33. B
34. A
35. A
36. B
37. A
38. False. You should take extra fluids to decrease the viscosity, no increase the viscosity
39. True
40. False. Albuterol sustained-release tablets should be protected from moisture. Tablets and syrup should be stored between 2 and 30 degrees C, inhalation albuterol should be stored between 15 and 30 degrees C.

41. False. You should not eat this type of diet while on theophylline because it decreases the theophylline level.
42. True
43. False. You should not alter dose or frequency of any form of albuterol without consulting with your primary care provider
44. False. Foods must be low in fat.
45. False. You should not exceed 12 inhalations in 24 hours.
46. True
47. True

CHAPTER 46

1. L
2. E
3. H
4. B
5. J
6. I
7. D
8. F
9. A
10. K
11. C
12. M
13. G
14. Mouth
15. Nasopharynx
16. Saliva
17. Lubricates
18. Protective
19. Digestion
20. Swallowing
21. Esophagus
22. Gastroesophageal
23. Peristaltic
24. Mucus
25. Parietal
26. Pepsin
27. Vitamin B_{12}
28. Pepsinogen
29. Gastric
30. Digestion
31. Absorption
32. Villi
33. Peristalsis

34. Brunner's
35. Pancreas
36. Digestive
37. Lipase
38. Electrolytes
39. Potassium
40. Lubricate
41. Absorption
42. Rectum
43. Internal
44. Sphincter
45. Metabolic
46. Carbohydrate
47. Lipid
48. Urea
49. Detoxification
50. Bile
51. Bile
52. Duodenum
53. Digestive juice
54. Enzymes
55. Bicarbonate
59. C
60. C
61. B
62. D
63. C

CHAPTER 47

16. False. The three responses are headaches, dizziness, and somnolence.
17. True.
18. True
19. False. It should be taken at least 30 minutes prior to meals.
20. False. It is classified as a category X drug, contraindicated during pregnancy.
21. False. Not antimuscarinics, but sucralfate (Carafate)
22. True
23. True
24. False. Other drugs must be administered at least 2 hours prior to the sucralfate to prevent drug-drug interactions.
25. True
26. False. The cations are magnesium, aluminum, sodium, and calcium. The anions are hydroxide, bicarbonate, citrate, carbonate, and phosphate.

27. True
28. True.
29. F
30. G
31. I
32. H
33. B
34. A
35. J
36. E
37. L
38. C
39. K
40. D
41. D
42. C
43. C
44. B

CHAPTER 48

10. Effectiveness of these agents depends on optimum fluid intake; they may cause obstruction if intake is poor.
11. Aspiration of oil droplets may result in lipid pneumonia.
12. The oil is very bland and may cause nausea. It is usually more palatable if chilled and given with fruit juices.
13. Loss of the enteric coat on the tablet will cause gastric irritation. Milk dissolves the coat.
14. Encopresis (fecal soiling) may be a symptom of chronic functional constipation.
15. Many medications have a side effect of constipation, and may be causing or exacerbating the problem. The client may be self-prescribing laxatives or enemas.
16. The medication is most effective when taken this way. The large volume of solution evacuates and cleanse the bowel.
17. Fever would suggest infectious diarrhea. Poor skin turgor and dry mucous membranes indicate dehydration.
18. A bland diet usually includes dairy products which are not recommended if the client is lactose intolerant.
19. This medication may have a side effect of drowsiness.
20. Lomotil contains atropine, which may cause problems for persons with glaucoma and/or prostate enlargement.

21. The administration of salicylates in the Pepto-Bismol to children with viral infection may lead to Reye's Syndrome.
22. Any systemic medications taken during pregnancy may have a possible effect on the fetus.
23. Sandostatin alters the secretion of insulin and glucagon.
24. D
25. C
26. A
27. C
28. B
29. B
30. D
31. F
32. C
33. A
34. E
35. D
36. A
37. C
38. B

CHAPTER 49

13. Skin, nasal hairs, eyelids, eyelashes, and mucous membranes
14. Fever, coughing, sneezing, vomiting, and excretory processes
15. Perspiration, tears, gastric juice, vaginal secretions, and saliva
16. Normal microorganisms that retard the colonization of other potentially harmful organisms. Escherichia coli
17. Neutrophils
18. Monocytes
19. Macrophages
20. Lymphokines
21. Mobile
22. Tissue
23. Blood
24. Clots
25. Temperature
26. Infected
27. Plasma
28. Tissue
29. Pathway
30. Enhance
31. Antibody-antigen

32. Phagocytes
33. B
34. Antigens
35. Complement
36. Polypeptides
37. Immune
38. Antibodies
39. Antigen
40. Decreases
41. Foreign
42. D
43. B
44. A

CHAPTER 50

7. mast cells; basophils
8. capillary permeability
9. antihistamines
10. anticholinergic
11. stimulation
12. hypersensitivity
13. slower

CHAPTER 51

6. Prostaglandin synthetase inhibitors (PSIs)
7. Nonprostaglandin synthetase inhibitors (non-PSIs)
8. Inflammation
9. Pain
10. Fever
11. Biosynthesis
12. Release
13. Trauma
14. Chronic inflammatory disease
15. PSIs
16. Other mechanisms
24. Cardiovascular
25. Arthritis
26. Dysmenorrhea
27. 1-3
28. 3-4
29. GI tract
30. Plasma proteins
31. Bile
32. Liver

33. Kidneys
34. 24
35. PG synthesis
36. 20-30
37. Menstrual; Uterine
42. A
43. B

CHAPTER 52

1. H
2. D
3. J
4. F
5. C
6. A
7. I
8. E
9. G
10. B
11. Cytotoxins
12. T-helper cell suppressors
13. Lymphocyte antibodies
14. Corticosteroids
15. Renal
16. Bone marrow grafts
17. 1-2
18. Less
19. Erythrocytes
20. Urine
21. Small intestine
22. Plasma proteins
23. Fat, liver
24. 19
25. Feces
26. Urine
27. Self-replication
28. DNA, RNA
29. Foreign
30. Cellular
31. Bone marrow
32. T-helper
33. Maturing
34. High
35. Hematologic
36. GI
37. Myelosuppression

38. Nausea and vomiting
39. Infection
40. Renal failure
41. Hepatotoxicity
42. Not recommended
43. Breast-feeding mothers
44. Direct contact
45. Toxic
46. Drug concentrations
47. Nephrotoxicity, hepatotoxicity
48. Oral
49. Subtherapeutic
50. Allograft
51. Aplastic
52. Acute
53. Cell-mediated
54. Antigens
55. Foreign antigens
56. Anaphylaxis
57. Chemical
58. "Flu-like"
59. Glomerular filtration rate
60. Skin test
61. Epinephrine
62. High-flow
63. Glucocorticoids
64. B
65. A
66. A
67. D
68. B

CHAPTER 53

6. GI tract
7. $1/2$ to $1 \, 1/2$ hours
8. 1 hour
9. placenta and blood-brain
10. liver
11. urine
12. retrovirus replication and DNA chain termination
13. monophosphate
14. triphosphate
15. Headaches, nausea, and insomnia
16. Macrocytic anemia

7. bone marrow
8. Myopathy
9. renal or hepatic
10. C
11. A
12. D

CHAPTER 54

13. enzymes
14. Lysis
16. abnormal
17. ribosomes
18. genetic
19. replication
21. Bind
22. permeability
23. metabolic
24. cell
26. RNA, DNA
31. E, H
32. C, F
33. A, G
34. B, D
35. B
36. A
37. D

CHAPTER 55

9. D
10. D
11. G
12. C
13. B
14. F
15. B
16. A
17. E
18. D
19. D
20. A
21. A
22. B
23. A
24. B
25. B

26. A
27. B
42. False. They should do this to prevent a photosensitivity reaction.
43. True
44. True
45. False. This is Stevens Johnson syndrome.
46. False. Neuromuscular blocking agents should not be taken with Cleocin for these reasons.
47. False. These are signs of cholestatic jaundice.
48. True.
49. False. Allergic reaction to penicillin is the most common.
50. False. IV vancomycin should be infused over 60–90 minutes to prevent this syndrome.
57. B
58. C
59. A
60. B
61. C

CHAPTER 56

9. NegGram
10. Furadantin
11. Hiprex
12. cystitis
13. Long term
14. DNA
15. carbohydrate
16. formaldehyde, Formaldehyde
17. liver
18. Breast feeding mothers
19. diabetic
20. Dehydration
21. Hepatic
22. anticoagulants
23. nalidixic
24. Antacids
25. gastric
26. Sulfa
27. alkalinize
28. N, F, M
29. N
30. N, F
31. M
32. N, F
33. N, F

34. F
35. N,F
36. F
37. F

CHAPTER 57

1. rapid
2. 1 to 2 hours; lengthened
3. genetically; faster
4. bactericidal; biosynthesis of component of cell wall
5. rapidly replicating; bacteriostatic, bactericidal; RNA synthesis
11. A
12. B
13. D
14. B

CHAPTER 58

21. thrush
22. imidazoles and triazoles
23. amphotericin B
24. flucytosine
25. 100 mcg/ml
26. ketoconazole and itraconazole
27. griseofulvin
28. sexual intercourse

CHAPTER 59

6. B
7. C
8. G
9. F
10. B
11. D
12. B
13. E
14. E
15. B
16. C
17. True
18. True
19. False. A decreased platelet count is an adverse effect of vidarabine.
20. False. Elderly clients are most susceptible to renal impairment.

21. False. Amantadine is also recommended as a prophylactic drug.
22. True
23. True
24. True
25. False. OSHA mandates disposed of unused portions of Acyclovir.
26. True
27. False. Interferons have immunoregulatory and antiviral properties.
28. True
29. True
30. False. Ribavarin is delivered via a small-particle aerosal generator.
31. True
32. True

CHAPTER 60

7. M
8. I
9. L
10. H
11. P
12. E
13. O
14. A
15. F
16. B
17. G
18. I
19. D
20. C
21. P
22. K
23. M
24. J
25. N
26. B
30. A
31. D
32. B
33. A
34. C
35. D
36. B
37. C

CHAPTER 61

1. C
2. G
3. H
4. J
5. I
6. A
7. F
8. B
9. D
0. E
1. 10
2. capacitation
3. erection of penis; orgasm
8. B, C
9. B
20. A, D
21. B, C

CHAPTER 62

8. infertility; Gn-Rh
9. FSH; LH
10. pulsatile; normal secretory patterns of the hypothalamus.
11. ovulation
12. estrogenic; nonestrogenic; hypothalamic-pituitary
axis; LH; FSH
13. endometriosis; uterine fibroids
14. stimulates; FSH; LH; desensitized; FSH; LH;
diminished
19. A
20. D
21. C
22. B

CHAPTER 63

7. D
8. M
9. N
10. M
11. M
12. T
26. False. It enhances the tendency for edema.
27. True
28. True
29. True

30. False. The three are : esters, 17-α alkalated, and
modified ring structure
31. True
32. False. Finasteride causes a decrease in the PSA
levels, even in the presence of prostatic cancer;
therefore this is not an effective screening tool in
this instance.
33. False. Severe effects are liver and cardiovascular
impairment and psychotic syndrome.

CHAPTER 64

15. D
16. F
17. G
18. A
19. C
20. H
21. B
22. I
23. J
24. E

CHAPTER 65

11. D
12. C
13. E
14. A
15. B
16. B
17. C
18. A
19. B
20. A
21. C
22. B
23. D

CHAPTER 66

17. A, B, C, D
18. A, B, C
19. A, C, D

CHAPTER 67

9. A, F
10. B, I
11. B, H
12. C, D, G

13. C, E, D	35. B
14. C, E	36. D
19. D	
20. C	**CHAPTER 68**
21. F	
22. A	22. A
23. A	23. C
24. E	24. B
25. G	25. C
26. B	
27. G	**CHAPTER 69**
28. F	
29. A	11. B
30. E	12. D
31. D	13. C
32. H	14. A
33. B	
34. C	

CHAPTER 70

```
C  O  E  E  I  M  F  D  Z  A  J  Q  Q  L  O  R  I  P  F  S
G  J  S  W  B  P  N  M  A  C  R  O  M  I  N  E  R  A  L  S
U  G  L  Z  D  W  V  D  C  E  Z  F  Y  S  Y  Z  T  A  K  E
I  B  Z  P  E  U  R  I  S  Y  D  Q  A  K  B  -  R  G  W  I
H  H  A  G  L  Y  C  O  G  E  N  G  D  T  S  E  Y  Y  R  R
W  F  G  N  B  N  C  F  Z  R  D  Q  H  O  N  V  M  R  S  O
S  C  O  T  U  U  N  K  D  B  X  V  L  I  P  I  D  M  E  L
X  E  L  C  L  T  S  F  P  D  C  U  M  I  S  K  T  E  Y  A
W  G  T  G  O  X  R  C  A  R  B  O  H  Y  D  R  A  T  E  C
A  I  S  I  S  K  L  I  L  L  R  X  Q  O  E  S  J  D  Y  O
K  M  Q  U  -  I  L  F  E  C  V  N  S  T  J  H  E  Z  N  L
N  C  A  F  R  V  C  V  I  N  G  D  W  R  T  F  M  C  X  I
C  Y  T  P  E  Z  I  M  V  H  T  R  Y  E  T  B  M  T  O  K
L  L  A  N  T  T  T  N  R  V  Q  S  J  S  U  U  D  D  C  O
D  J  W  G  A  E  K  P  V  W  I  S  P  C  F  U  V  W  E  P
T  E  L  M  W  W  W  N  V  C  D  A  U  I  M  V  O  E  G  E
G  J  I  N  G  Z  Z  I  M  J  B  B  P  C  Q  K  O  O  Z  N
B  N  D  C  B  B  V  I  Z  V  F  S  M  A  D  N  A  Y  Q
S  Y  K  K  R  R  O  B  A  I  T  U  O  A  W  W  T  F  I  A
C  W  Q  I  A  L  B  T  A  G  L  R  V  D  O  S  W  I  M  V
```

1. calorie		8. nutrients
2. carbohydrate		9. vitamins
3. fat-soluble vitamins		10. RDA
4. glucose		11. water soluble
5. glycogen		12. water
6. kilocalories		13. macrominerals
7. lipid		14. microminerals

CHAPTER 71

1. C, G, I, N, P, S
2. E, H, K O, T
3. A, D, J, M, R
4. B, F, L, Q
5. B, E, H, J, K, L
6. B, G, I, L
7. B, C, L
8. A, B, D, E, F, H, L
9. Chronic Vitamin A
0. Chronic Vitamin D
1. Acute Vitamin D
2. Acute Vitamin A
7. False. Vitamin A
8. True
9. False. Vitamin K
0. True
1. False. Hypermagnesemia
2. False. renal failure
3. False. Vitamin K
4. C
5. B
6. D
7. B

CHAPTER 72

15. G
16. D
17. I
18. H
19. J
20. A
21. F
22. K
23. B
24. E
25. C
37. C
38. A
39. D
40. C

CHAPTER 73

14. A
15. B

16. A
17. B
18. B
19. B
20. A
21. B
22. B
23. A
24. A
25. B
26. A
27. B
28. B
29. B

CHAPTER 74

1. B
2. D
3. A
4. C
7. albumin
8. bicarbonate
9. colloid
10. crystalloid
11. dextran
12. granulocytes
13. hypermagnesemia
14. hyperosmolar
15. hypertonic
16. hypokalemia
17. hyponatremia
18. hypotonic
19. isotonic
20. oncotic
21. osmolality
22. osmosis

CHAPTER 75

1. anabolism
2. anthropometric
3. aspiration
4. blenderized
5. carbohydrates
6. enteral
7. Glucerna

8. lipids
9. macrominerals
10. Meritene
11. modular
12. polymeric
13. Procalamine
14. proteins
19. D
20. A

CHAPTER 76

13. A, D
14. B
15. A
16. A, B
17. A
18. A, B
19. B, E
20. E
21. C
22. S
23. C
24. C
25. S
26. C
27. S